Writing Cancer

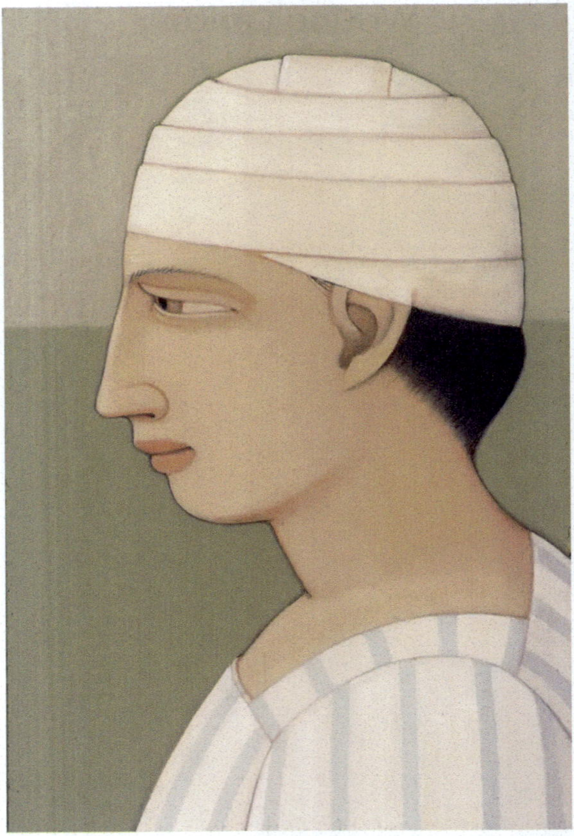

'Portrait: Wrapped Head' by Andrew Stevovich. Oil on linen, 1988. Private collection. Reproduced with permission

Ad A. Kaptein • Brian M. Hughes

Writing Cancer

Literary Explorations of a Timeless Disease

palgrave
macmillan

Ad A. Kaptein
Medical Psychology
Leiden University Medical Center
Leiden, The Netherlands

Brian M. Hughes
School of Psychology
University of Galway
Galway, Ireland

ISBN 978-981-95-6500-9 ISBN 978-981-95-6501-6 (eBook)
https://doi.org/10.1007/978-981-95-6501-6

This Palgrave Macmillan imprint is published by the registered company Springer Nature Singapore Pte Ltd.
The registered company address is: 152 Beach Road, #21-01/04 Gateway East, Singapore 189721, Singapore

ALSO BY AD A. KAPTEIN

Behavioural Medicine: Psychological Treatment of Somatic Disorders
Psychology in Medicine
Respiratory Disorders and Behavioral Medicine
Health Psychology

ALSO BY BRIAN HUGHES

Conceptual and Historical Issues in Psychology
Rethinking Psychology: Good Science, Bad Science, Pseudoscience
Psychology in Crisis
The Psychology of Brexit: From Psychodrama to Behavioural Science
A Conceptual History of Psychology: The Mind Through Time
Psychology's Quiet Conservatism: How a Supposedly Woke Science Promotes Capitalism and Protects Privilege

Acknowledgements

For a number of years, the *British Medical Journal* carried a column called 'Between the Lines' in which Theodore Dalrymple discussed novels about illness. His columns were an inspiration for one of us—namely, Ad—to write a number of articles on this theme of literature and medicine. This theme turned out also to be attractive for *Cicero*, Leiden University Medical Centre's (LUMC) monthly magazine, who compiled and published a number of these articles under the title *Helende Woorden* ('Healing Words'). Since 2019, the magazine *Medische Oncologie* carried similar columns by Ad, all written in Dutch, in which he discussed works of literature that had cancer as a central theme. The present volume is prompted by and largely derived from these original columns.

The second of us—namely, Brian—was invited to take Ad's columns as prompts to revisit, re-evaluate, and re-write all the content, taking account of his own experience and expertise in the field of (critical) health psychology, and adding new insights from physiology and cultural studies. Ad and Brian are longstanding collaborators, and this new venture stimulated much energetic discussion. As such, the present volume is more than a mere translation; it is a reimagining and refashioning of a newly co-authored product.

Sincere thanks to Marion Duval at Palgrave Macmillan and to Keerthana Ramalingam for their valuable support. Many thanks to Freek

Bouricius for offering a foothold in *Medische Oncologie*. Jan Schoones, of the Walaeus Library, LUMC, was a tireless expert in collecting literature about being ill. Jos Leenes and Antoine Rijnders, Parnassia group librarians, were critical readers and found more obscure sources from books and articles. Frans Meulenberg was a reader and encouraged the writing from the very beginning, and later on, Pim van der Meer and Fleur Fisher also fulfilled this role. Their verdict was always critical and constructive. Emma Wilson translated Ad's Dutch text into English. Michael Murray, Keele University, offered editorial help in the early phases of the book. Lucia Snoei carried over her design from the cover of *Helende Woorden* to *Kanker Schrijven*. Many thanks to Ton van Poelgeest and Herman Masthoff, of Elmar Publishers, Delft, for their care in the original publication of *Kanker Schrijven*. Thanks also to the sponsors who supported the authors' prior research and publication.

We also want to thank our friends and families for all their social support. Brian wishes especially to thank Marguerite, Louis, and Annie. Ad thanks Carla.

This book is intended for physicians and other healthcare providers who deal with persons with cancer—and possibly, also, for those dealing with other conditions. The book may also be of interest to researchers and teachers in literary studies in the medical, psychological, and related fields. It would be great if they encouraged their students to read at least one of the literary works discussed on the succeeding pages.

Ad and Brian
Leiden and Galway
February 2026

Contents

1

Having Cancer

1.1 Science, Charity, and Medicine

Having completed his initial studies at Barcelona's School of Fine Arts, Pablo Picasso was just 15 years old when he produced one of his most intriguing early paintings. The scene depicts an ill young woman lying in bed, attended to by a bearded man in a black suit. A nun stands nearby, presenting the woman with a drink and holding a little girl in her arms. Picasso was a gifted but methodical artist: he asked his own father to pose as the model for the bearded man, and based the nun on a passer-by he had met one day on the street. For the sick woman, Picasso painted an image resembling his sister Conchita, who herself had died from diphtheria two years previously, aged just seven; tragically, Picasso's family were not wealthy enough to avail of what was then a brand new treatment for diphtheria, one of several medical breakthroughs to attract growing public attention as the twentieth century beckoned. In his painting, Picasso portrayed the young woman as having pale skin, suggesting an affliction with tuberculosis.

It is striking that Picasso entitled this work *Ciencia y Caridad*, or 'Science and Charity.' Historically, medical care was not always seen as something to be infused with science, and it was not always appreciated that medicine

A. A. Kaptein, B. M. Hughes, *Writing Cancer*,
https://doi.org/10.1007/978-981-95-6501-6_1

might gain—or perhaps lose—from a scientific approach. Viewing this painting today, most medical students usually say without hesitating that the bearded man is a *doctor*, and, further, that this *doctor* is the person responsible for looking after the patient. But the bearded man in this painting does not even look at the young woman, instead focusing on measuring her pulse. For her part, the woman shares meaningful eye contact with the nun and the child, broadening our appreciation of what it really means to be 'looked after.' On the left, science. On the right, perhaps, charity.

Art historians will usually point out that Picasso has allowed light to fall upon the nun and the child while the doctor sits in relative shade, and that the mirror above the patient's head is covered by a black cloth, a symbol of impending death. As such, in the artist's view, the scientific approach alone might not have all the answers.

It can be helpful to summarise this painting by distinguishing the 'biomedical' from the 'psychological'. Traditionally framed, the so-called biomedical model translates disease experiences into observable phenomena, focusing on 'that which can be measured' rather than on that which is truly important. Data are derived from objective indices, such as the patient's pulse; the patient's own views of their symptoms, their disease state, and especially their treatment, are seen as not really medically relevant. When viewed scientifically this way, being ill is something for doctors to describe, rather than for patients to ponder.

By contrast, a psychological approach to illness will attempt to approach illness as something patients (certainly) live through, rather than (potentially) die from. The psychological dimensions of disease—the combined elements of the entire experience of being sick—are seen as being just as integral to medical care as all its biomedical aspects.

A classic depiction of the biomedical model is discussed by Kaplan (1990). It considers five sets of determinants of tissue or organ pathology (namely, complications at birth, illness, ageing, genetic predisposition, and accidents) which are said to be responsible for precipitating symptoms and illnesses, and which—all going well, presumably—can successfully be addressed using 'medical' intervention. Notably, of the various disease determinants included, none encompass societal, social, or behavioural factors. This is despite the fact that many such factors—for example, poverty—are among the most reliable statistical predictors of a person's likelihood of future illness.

Nonetheless, the biomedical model is certainly useful when it comes to acute conditions, such as appendicitis or a broken leg. Indeed, in such contexts, it can be truly life-saving. However, for many illness scenarios, particularly those relating to oncology, it quickly becomes clear that the biomedical approach has many shortcomings. For one thing, its final step—'decreased pathology'—is very often far from the end of the care journey for people with cancer. In cancer, the primary concern is often more the *quality* of life than its quantity, and for most patients in this situation, medical care can only reasonably be evaluated in these terms. While the phrase 'quality of life' can itself mean different things to different people, as we will discuss below, in health research it is often used to refer to the effects of diseases and treatments *as they are experienced* by patients. The subjective experience of the individual is key.

We have always observed that medical students—even those quite advanced in their studies—typically become defensive when discussing Picasso's *Ciencia y Caridad,* questioning why the nun, the child, and their eye contact with the patient should get all this attention. The qualitative aspects of medical care are all very well, they say, but the scientifically informed input of the doctor is surely essential for the patient's eventual well-being. But the message of the painting is not that the doctor is somehow irrelevant, or that biomedical concerns should be ignored. Instead, Picasso's depiction of medicine is inclusive. It shows how medicine encompasses more than just biomedical science alone; it asserts that 'charity'—or what we might refer to today as 'psychosocial care'—is also integral.

This combination of 'biomedical' and 'psychosocial' forms the basis of what has become known as the biopsychosocial model of health and illness. The biopsychosocial model was first famously formulated by American psychiatrist George Engel in 1977, in a paper entitled *The need for a new medical model: A challenge for biomedicine* (see also Brody 1973). The essence of the approach can be discerned quickly: biomedical processes that lead to changes in tissues, organs, and the nervous system, themselves produce changes in a person's perceptions and behaviour—in other words, in their *experiences.* These changes in turn exert knock-on effects on the person's interactions with other individuals and with wider society. The impact of the 'bio' on both 'psycho' and 'social' is clear.

However, crucially, the effects in Engel's model flow in both directions: wider social and cultural conditions themselves impact upon a person's perceptions and behaviours, and these perceptions and behaviours themselves impact upon their personal well-being. Such impacts can be direct or indirect. Direct impacts can result from neurological and psychophysiological processes, such as when chronic life stress leads to elevated blood pressure or the slow denigration of immune function. But indirect impacts are just as—or even more—important. These arise as a result of a person's choices and circumstances, such as their smoking or self-care habits, their social exclusion from health services, or a level of material impoverishment that leads to, for example, poor nutrition. Both direct and indirect impacts ensure that the cultural interacts with the cellular: biological outcomes are moderated by perception and behaviour, which themselves are intertwined with social conditions. Thus the flow of influence across bio, psycho, and social is bidirectional. All three aspects operate simultaneously and are interrelated.

For Engel, these relationships explain why disintegrating societies (e.g., Russia after 1990) become characterised by diminished life expectancies. In such places, inherent social instability leads to widespread psychological distress and an upsurge in health-damaging activities, such as increased levels of alcohol use. These shifts eventually translate into higher rates of physical illnesses, such as cancer, in the general population.

There have certainly been many criticisms of what Engel proposed. For example, while more expansive than traditional biomedicine, the biopsychosocial framing still generally fails to take account of the broader experiential, critical, and sociopolitical realities of cancer. The effort to incorporate psychological and social dimensions appears restricted to individual perspectives, thereby maintaining a focus on the subjective—on individual experiences within social contexts, rather than on, say, societal impacts on disease. The biopsychosocial approach emphasises the way personal multifaceted psychologies intertwine with personal experiences of cancer, but it rarely directly enquires about the role of political and economic systems in creating the type of toxic environments in which cancer is far more likely to strike some human beings more than others. Indeed, because of this focus on apolitical subjectivity, the biopsychosocial model could be said to play its own part in perpetuating a victim-blaming narrative convenient to elites, where diseases such as cancer are cast not as grand societal or political challenges, but as personal plights addressable primarily through person-level intervention (cf., Hughes 2025).

Moreover, several attempts to recast the biopsychosocial model have proven to be especially controversial (frequently, it has to be said, because of a failure to recognise that Engel's model explicitly *includes*, rather *rejects*, traditional biomedical processes). But, all that being said, that is not the point here. What is important is that the biopsychosocial approach recognises—in fact, it proclaims—that 'being ill' is more than just being ill in one, biomedical, sense; a proclamation that serves as the core message of this introductory chapter, and indeed of this book as a whole.

Our ethos is easy to express: cancer is more than just the growth of malignant cells; therefore, the effects of medical care on people with cancer should be measured by more than just the assessment of the number or nature of such cells. This principle is increasingly acknowledged in modern medicine by both academics and practitioners. Whether explicitly or implicitly, the biopsychosocial ethos is endorsed by the majority of major medical journals, and not just journals of public health or psychology. These days, every single issue of the *Journal of Clinical Oncology*, for example, will carry at least one article that gives direct attention to biopsychosocial concepts.

1.2 From Theoretical Models to the Clinic

Such theoretical models can sometimes appear abstract, but they have practical significance too.

Treating cancer within a biopsychosocial framework requires us to take seriously the various beliefs a patient will have regarding their condition, including their understanding of how they became ill in the first place and how behavioural and social factors might ultimately impact on their well-being. This is not to suggest that psychological influences actually *cause* cancers, but merely to point out that, once illness has struck, behavioural and attitudinal factors are essential to ensuring that the patient engages in the type of lifestyle changes needed to enhance their health over time. Securing patient commitment is central to the success of many therapies, but also to that of diagnoses. Also important is to ensure that a patient maintains an authentic social existence while ill, and to allow their social system to play as large a role as possible in supporting their self-management. Taking account of what is important to patients is necessary for effective treatment decisions.

Throughout this book, we will examine how a diverse set of authors have written about their experiences of having cancer. We will use their accounts to consider their perceptions of the psychological, the biological, and the social. We will ask a number of questions. What attributions did the writers make regarding their illnesses? How did these attributions influence their reactions and their self-management behaviours? What kind of self-regulation or self-management skills—if any—did they exhibit? Overall, we will explore what lessons we can draw from the way these authors have been *writing cancer*.

1.3 Managing the Self

Decades ago, the idea that people with cancer should somehow *manage themselves* was one that raised many a clinician's eyebrow. But the importance of self-management is widely accepted. It is seen as a valuable—and fundamentally biopsychosocial—component of modern cancer care, aimed at achieving the best possible quality of life for patients (Boland et al. 2018; Caminiti et al. 2021; Cuthbert et al. 2019; Haase et al. 2021). It is worth noting that self-management only partially involves obtaining or asking for information; instead, a patient's focus is usually on trying to derive personal meaning from cancer and its treatment. As such, providing so-called patient education might ultimately prove of limited use in supporting a patient's self-management efforts (this is why, in an article about adherence to oral targeted therapy, we used a somewhat provocative subtitle—"*We don't need no education*"—to emphasise the desirability of a broader approach; Kaptein et al. 2021). Indeed, the very idea that a patient should 'adhere to' or 'comply with' physician instructions itself suggests an unwarranted primacy of the biomedical, overlooking those psychological and social dimensions that affect the patient's experience of illness and recovery. What is needed, surely, is not adherence or compliance. What is needed is 'collaboration'—between patient and doctor (and, indeed, others).

In our view, self-management by people with cancer is best promoted by connecting with what the patient thinks, feels, and experiences, taking full account of the meanings that the patient gives to their disease. In the following chapters, we will focus on one particular method with which (some) patients have created such meanings: the creative and expressive arts. In turn, we will explore the potential of literature (as well as of films, music, and paintings) as a means of helping patients to live with their cancer by illustrating ways in which self-management can constructively be achieved. In short, we will discuss how creative literature can provide powerful first-person perspectives on the lived experience of having cancer, and how such literature produces shareable meanings, in accessible forms, that readers can then use to pursue their own existential goals.

1.4 Quality of Life

Promoting self-management equates to the promotion of quality of life. Although references to 'quality of life' appeared in the social science literature since at least the 1920s, it was not until the 1960s that the physician J. R. Elkington (1966) introduced it to the medical literature, in a landmark editorial in the *Annals of Internal Medicine*. In this piece, Elkington considered the needs of an 88-year-old woman he had recently visited, on her birthday. Wondering what medical care could best contribute to people like her, he concluded: "improve quality of life."

Interest in how physicians could usefully *measure* this quality of life began to grow. A number of psychometric questionnaires were developed, some focusing on generic life quality, others on the quality of life of people with specific diseases. Academic journals dedicated to these topics began to appear, many under the auspices of scientific or professional organisations. Several continue to thrive today: examples relating to cancer include the journals *Quality of Life Research*, *Psycho-Oncology*, and *Supportive Care in Cancer*. Quality of life is also extensively discussed in generic cancer journals and in journals in the fields of behavioural medicine, medical psychology, and health psychology. Likewise, quality of life is commonly measured as a key outcome in research examining the effects of cancer and its medical management.

A study by Detmar et al. (2002) was one of the first in the field to explore quality of life of patients with cancer. The core aim of the research was to study the effects of complaints monitoring and self-management on patients' quality of life. An important conclusion of the authors was that "incorporating standard health-related quality of life (HRQL) assessments in daily oncology practice facilitates the discussion of HRQL issues and can heighten physicians' awareness of their patients' HRQL" (p. 3027). As such, the very process of attempting to record a patient's quality of life can help doctors to better appreciate the life perspectives of the people under their care.

A more recently developed but related concept is 'patient-reported outcome', or PRO. This concept also reflects the patient's perception of the process of medical treatment, as well as its effects. It has proven so useful as to have yielded its own dedicated journal, the *Journal of Patient-Reported Outcomes* (established in 2017).

Crucially, patients' judgements about the nature and effects of medical treatment do not always reflect those of their physicians. A doctor's evaluations of side effects, even when measured using internationally accepted criteria, will often deviate sharply from a patient's own judgement of their symptoms and quality of life (see, for example, Atkinson et al. 2019, 2020; Fares et al. 2018). This is important because there is some evidence to suggest that symptom monitoring appears to be associated with meaningfully improved treatment outcomes, including, in some cases, better survival rates (see Basch et al. 2020). A recent study by Hui et al. (2022), for example, found that lung cancer or prostate cancer patients whose quality of life was monitored had longer survival than patients in a control group whose quality of life was not tracked. Even stronger empirical support for the importance of examining the voice of the patient was recently published in a systematic review and meta-analysis of studies on patient-reported outcomes (PROs) as prognostic indicators for overall survival in cancer: it was found that PROs offer independent prognostic information for cancer survival (Huang et al. 2025). This provides further justification for considering patients' perceptions of illness as deserving of careful study.

Of course, if monitoring patients' experiences is helpful, it stands to reason that seeking to enhance those experiences might also produce critical benefits. Interventions that aim to modify a patient's perceptions of their illness and its treatment may well help to enhance their quality of life, including in ways that, in turn, enhance the outcomes of medical treatment. Such interventions can, in theory, assist patients to formulate more adaptive and constructive attitudes to their plight: to the challenges of being ill, to their experiences of (and thus engagement with) medical treatment, and to the various reactions to their disease that they encounter in social contexts. Unsurprisingly, research into such interventions is vast. Reviewing the field, Rodin et al. (2020) sought to identify psychological interventions that yield especially positive outcomes in people with cancer. They found that many such interventions help in reducing patients' depression, anxiety, and distress, and above all, in increasing their overall quality of life. Some of the most effective interventions produce these benefits by helping patients to cultivate a personal sense of meaning, improvement, and enrichment of social existence, and by decreasing their perceived limitations in physical activity (Rodin et al. 2020). Overall, formal reviews and meta-analyses suggest that, when used with people with cancer, these interventions are generally positive for patients, helping to enhance quality of life and to promote adaptive coping behaviour (e.g., Richardson et al. 2017, 2019).

1.5 Art as Medicine

When Picasso painted *Ciencia y Caridad*, he did not wish to merely record a visual image of the scene for posterity, as if pre-empting the use of photography. His purpose was much more than that. He wanted to produce *art*.

In many ways, artistic creativity is a profoundly psychological endeavour. Whatever their chosen genre, all artists are dedicated to eliciting fresh experiences in the minds of their readers, their viewers, or their listeners. The purpose of art is to *change* those who consume it, to produce new perspectives on human experience, to modify what it is that people feel, both emotionally and cognitively.

As such, when authors write creatively about cancer, in works of either fiction or non-fiction, their purpose is to provoke a psychological change in the minds of their readers. In this way, literature can then serve as its own form of psychosocial intervention: something that can help a person with cancer to reframe their understanding of what their illness and its treatment will bring, and how they might choose to respond. Something, in other words, that can, in a profound manner, influence the quality of their lives.

Literature is not the only art form in which cancer can be depicted. Films, music, and paintings (and to a lesser extent, dance, drama, and sculpture) have also been used to portray a variety of cognitive and emotional responses to cancer. Several researchers have explored how these different genres have been, or can be, deployed in therapeutic ways—whether through bibliotherapy, expressive writing, watching (or even making) films, listening to music, performing music, or viewing paintings—a theme we examine in the next chapter. For now, we can reflect on the fact that using art to cultivate a sense of meaning from suffering fits broadly into the biopsychosocial approach to healthcare. In our view, art can therefore enrich medicine in many ways, by enhancing the well-being of patients and their caregivers. (It can even deepen the job satisfaction of healthcare professionals.)

This rapid academic and clinical growth has been accompanied with, and stimulated by, the development of theoretical frameworks, clinical interventions, and educational programmes in fields such as health psychology, health humanities, medical humanities, and literature and medicine. These domains are now increasingly embedded in the curricula of medical, psychological, and healthcare training programmes. At the centre of this interdisciplinary field lies the concept of the *illness narrative*, often defined as "autobiographical accounts of illness spoken or written by patients" (Jurecic 2012, p. 2). Illness narratives encapsulate the subjective experience of symptoms and the personal, social, and professional responses to those symptoms.

Illness narratives provide a conceptual and methodological foundation for investigating how individuals write about illness, especially cancer. From a medical sociology perspective, Arthur Frank (1995) extended previous models by proposing distinct classes of illness narrative, such as *restitution chaos*, and *quest* (we will return to Frank's ideas later). In this book, we examine 30 examples of literature about cancer to investigate how these three narrative types manifest. Our analysis supports Frank's observation that in any illness all three narrative types often coexist—"alternatively and repeatedly…like patterns in a kaleidoscope" (1995, p. 76). Clinically, each narrative type suggests different forms of psychosocial intervention: from information provision in restitution narratives to existential therapy in chaos narratives, to self-management support in quest narratives (Bauereiss et al. 2018; Gu et al. 2024; de Sain et al. 2025).

From a cultural anthropological standpoint, the psychiatrist Arthur Kleinman famously promoted the notion of 'explanatory models', stories that people tell themselves, their loved ones, and their healthcare providers about their physical states and illnesses (whether 'objectively' correct or not). Kleinman (1988) emphasises that such stories are "justifications for practical action" rather than abstract theories (p. 121). Explanatory models provide insight into patients' attributions about their cancer, which may well be important for informing how communication and care can be better tailored to produce improved outcomes (e.g., Kang et al. 2025). In literary terms, they are narrative frameworks that often diverge sharply from biomedical interpretations.

From health psychology, the Common Sense Model (CSM) offers a cognitive framework for understanding how individuals perceive illness in terms of its causes, consequences, timeline, control, and identity (Leventhal et al. 2016). These perceptions are said to shape coping behaviour and to thereby influence multiple health outcomes, including quality of life (e.g., Zhang et al. 2024).

Illness perceptions, explanatory models, and illness narratives thus form a trifecta of overlapping yet distinct frameworks offering conceptual and clinical tools potentially applicable in cancer care. However, despite their growing scholarly recognition, discussions of illness narratives often remain marginalised in biomedical contexts. Medical students are frequently taught in ways that lead them to consider patient narratives as subjective, unscientific, or even distracting; because of implicit norms that devalue patient perspectives that comprise what has been termed the *hidden curriculum* of medical training (Lawrence et al. 2018). As we will see, resistance to illness narrative is not necessarily limited to medicine. In literary criticism, there can often emerge considerable scepticism regarding whether patient stories should be taken at face value. Jurecic (2012) argues that the field is dominated by a "hermeneutics of suspicion" that perceives such texts as (medically) unreliable and naïve. Another type of resistance comes from the proponents of narrative medicine themselves. While many academics aim to integrate patient stories into clinical care (e.g., Charon 2010), critics argue that doing so risks *appropriating* patients' narratives for biomedical ends. O'Mahony (2013), for example, considers such appropriation "spiritually arrogant and potentially harmful" (p. 614; cf., Florijn et al. 2019; Strawson 2004).

1.6 Medical and Health Humanities

Efforts to create space for patients' stories within academia and clinical practice have led to the emergence of interdisciplinary fields such as *medical humanities* and *health humanities*. These domains use literature, philosophy, history, and ethics to explore the human experience of illness and caregiving (Bleakley 2015). They encompass diverse disciplines, including medical psychology, sociology, nursing, anthropology, literary studies, and behavioural sciences. Journals such as *Medical Humanities* and *Journal of Medical Humanities* support the development of this field, as do recent monographs and edited volumes (e.g., Jones and Pachucki 2022; Klugman and Lamb 2019; Crawford et al. 2015). (The term *health humanities* has especially gained among social scientists seeking to move beyond the biomedical framing implicit in the term "medical humanities"; e.g., Jones et al. 2017).

A central question, both scientific and political, concerns the effectiveness of health humanities approaches. Why invest time teaching medical trainees about narrative-, literature-, or art-based methods when core biomedical subjects already demand significant space in the curriculum? In response, a growing body of empirical research has documented several improvements in communication, psychological well-being, treatment adherence, and quality of life following health humanities interventions (e.g., Bone et al. 2024; Ousager and Johannessen 2010; Sonke et al. 2025). Nonetheless, resistance remains. A recent critique in *Physics of Life Reviews* (Skov and Nadal 2025) questioned the methodological rigour of many such studies. However, extensive rebuttals (e.g.,

Clift and Grebosz-Haring 2025; Howlin 2025) and systematic reviews continue to underscore the benefits of health humanities for health (see also Fancourt 2026).

As a consequence, the integration of health humanities into medical education has become relatively well established. Numerous scholarly works provide comprehensive overviews of practices in this area (e.g., Crawford et al. 2015; Klugman and Lamb 2019). An illustrative example from our own educational practice may serve to concretise the utility of such approaches in a medical school context. In one such class, one of us (A.A.K.) introduced medical students to illness narratives, inviting them to engage with literary (novels and poetry), visual (film and painting), and biomedical texts. The students also conducted interviews with patients living with a particular disease, which they then synthesised into a comprehensive manuscript analysing the patients' illness narratives. The pedagogical outcomes of these practices were promising: several students succeeded in publishing their work (Kaptein et al. 2012, *Storying Stories, Medical Education Development*). This example underscores both the feasibility and the scholarly merit of incorporating health humanities ideas into medical education (cf. El-Jawahri et al. 2020).

1.7 Fulfilling the Potential of 'Meaning'

Psychologist Howard Leventhal has contributed a variety of ideas to the field of health psychology, including major theories about the cognitive and emotional mechanisms that shape how patients cope with illness and how clinical practitioners formulate their opinions. Leventhal's contributions have proven especially durable, having highlighted the importance of 'meaning making' in clinical care (e.g., Leventhal 2019).

Potentially, such theories, models, and methods help us to understand not only how patients derive their own personal 'meanings' of illness, and the resultant 'coping' responses, but also how such meaning and coping might be influenced, through intervention, to help enhance patients' quality of life. They draw on broad theoretical approaches from fields such as sociology, psychology, and anthropology. But, as outlined above, medical students and healthcare professionals are often disinclined to spend time exploring, or even thinking about, such subject areas. For many of these physicians, talk of patients' stories, narratives, or explanatory models is just chatter and noise, something akin to the intrusion of anecdote into science.

But doctors were not always like this. Almost a century ago, the illustrious physician Francis Weld Peabody, remembered today largely for his research into typhoid fever and polio, offered an especially discerning observation. With great foresight, he beautifully described the purpose of medicine in an essay entitled 'The care of the patient' (1927), reprinted in *JAMA* in 2009:

> The good physician knows his patients through and through, and his knowledge is bought dearly. Time, sympathy and understanding must be lavishly dispensed, but the reward is to be found in that personal bond which forms the greatest satisfaction of the practice of medicine. One of the essential qualities of the clinician is interest in humanity, for the secret of the care of the patient is in caring for the patient. (p. 882)

Despite the volume of academic work that has been completed on the human experience of illness, this 'interest in humanity'—in fact, the very notion of 'humanity' itself—is often ignored in modern medicine.

Its re-introduction—in the form of the fields of 'medical humanities' and 'health humanities'—is what we discuss next.

References

Atkinson, T. M., C. E. Schwartz, L. Goldstein, I. Garcia, D. F. Storfer, Y. Li, J. Zhang, B. H. Bochner, B. D. Rapkin, et al. 2019. Perceptions of response burden associated with completion of patient-reported outcome assessments in oncology. *Value in Health* 22:225–230.

Atkinson, T. M., A. C. Dueck, D. V. Satele, G. Thanarajasingam, J. M. Lafky, J. A. Sloan, and E. Basch. 2020. Clinician vs patient reporting of baseline and postbaseline symptoms for adverse event assessment in cancer clinical trials. *JAMA Oncology* 6:437–439.

Basch, E., L. Wilfong, and D. Schrag. 2020. Adding patient-reported outcomes to medicare's oncology value-based payment model. *JAMA* 323:213–214.

Bauereiss, N., S. Obermaier, S. E. Özünal, and H. Baumeister. 2018. Effects of existential interventions on spiritual, psychological, and physical well-being in adult patients with cancer: Systematic review and meta-analysis of randomized controlled trials. *Psycho-Oncology* 27:2531–2545.

Bleakley, A. 2015. *Medical humanities and medical education*. London: Routledge.

Boland, L., K. Bennett, and D. Connolly. 2018. Self-management interventions for cancer survivors: A systematic review. *Supportive Care in Cancer* 26:1585–1595.

Bone, J. K., D. Fancourt, J. K. Sonke, and F. Bu. 2024. Participatory and receptive arts engagement in older adults: Associations with cognition over a seven-year period. *Creativity Research Journal* 36:436–450.

Brody, H. 1973. The systems view of man: Implications for medicine, science, and ethics. *Perspectives in Biology and Medicine* 17:71–92.

Caminiti, C., M. A. Annunziata, C. Verusio, C. Pinto, M. Airoldi, et al. 2021. Effectiveness of a psychosocial care quality improvement strategy to address quality of life in patients with cancer. *JAMA Network Open* 4:1–14.

Charon, R. 2010. Calculating the contributions of Humanities to medical practice – motives, methods, and metrics. *Academic Medicine* 85:935–937.

Clift, S., and K. Grebosz-Haring. 2025. The need for a critical perspective on arts and health research and reviews. Comment on "Can arts-based interventions improve health? A conceptual and methodological critique" by Martin Skov and Marcos Nadal. *Physics of Life Reviews* 54:116–119.

Crawford, P., B. Brown, C. Baker, V. Tischler, and B. Abrams, eds. 2015. *Health humanities*. London: Palgrave.

Cuthbert, C. A., J. F. Farragher, B. R. Hemmelgarn, Q. Ding, G. P. McKinnon, and W. Y. Cheung. 2019. Self-management interventions for cancer survivors: A systematic review and evaluation of intervention content and theories. *Psycho-Oncology* 28:2119–2140.

Detmar, S. B., M. J. Muller, J. H. Schornagel, L. D. V. Wever, and N. K. Aaronson. 2002. Health-related quality-of-life assessments and patient-physician communication. *JAMA* 288:3027–3034.

El-Jawahri, A., D. Forst, A. Fenech, K. O. Brenner, A. L. Jankowski, L. Waldman, I. Sereno, R. Nipp, J. A. Greer, L. Traeger, V. Jackson, and J. Temel. 2020. Relationship between perceptions of treatment goals and psychological distress in patients with advanced cancer. *Journal of the National Comprehensive Cancer Network* 18:849–855.

Elkington, J. R. 1966. Medicine and the quality of life. *Annals of Internal Medicine* 64:711–714.

Fancourt, D. 2026. *Art cure: The science of how the arts transform our health*. Cornerstone Press.

Fares, C. M., T. J. Williamson, M. K. Theisen, A. Cummings, K. Bornazyan, M. L. Carroll, A. L. Stanton, and E. B. Garon. 2018. Low concordance of patient-reported outcomes with clinical and clinical trial documentation. *Journal of Clinical Oncology* 2:1–12.

Florijn, B. W., H. van der Graaf, J. W. Schoones, and A. A. Kaptein. 2019. Narrative medicine: A comparison of terminal cancer patients' stories from a Dutch hospice with those of Anatole Broyard and Christopher Hitchens. *Death Studies* 43:570–581.

Frank, A. W. 1995. *The wounded storyteller. Body, illness, and ethics*. Chicago: The University of Chicago Press.

Gu, X., X. Shen, J. R. Zhou, J. H. Chu, and L. Jiang. 2024. The effects of common-sense model interventions on cancer patients. A systematic review. *Medicine* 103:17 (e37777).

Haase, K. R., S. Sattar, S. Hall, B. McLean, A. Wills, et al. 2021. Systematic review of self-management interventions for older adults with cancer. *Psycho-Oncology* 30:989–1008.

Howlin, C. 2025. There is more to arts than neural mechanisms: A critique of evidence dismissal in arts and health: Comment on "Can arts-based interventions improve health? A conceptual and methodological critique" by Martin Skov and Marcos Nadal. *Physics of Life Reviews* 54:89–91.

Huang, R. S., D. Chen, A. Benour, R. Cortez, A. Mihalache, C. Johnny, A. Bezjak, R. A. Olson, and S. Raman. 2025. Patient-reported outcomes as prognostic indicators for overall survival in cancer – a systematic review and meta-analysis. *JAMA Oncology*. https://doi.org/10.1001/jamaoncol.2025.3153, in press 11 September 2025.

Hughes, B. M. 2025. *Psychology's Quiet Conservatism: How a Supposedly Woke Science Promotes Capitalism and Protects Privilege*. Cham, Switzerland: Palgrave Macmillan.

Hui, D., A. K. Darke, K. A. Guthrie, I. M. Subbiah, J. M. Unger, D. L. Hershman, R. S. Krouse, M. Bakitas, and M. A. O'Rourke. 2022. Association between health-related quality of life and progression-free survival in patients with advanced cancer: A secondary analysis of SWOG clinical trials. *JCO Oncology Practice* 18:e442–e451.

Jones, T., and K. Pachucki, eds. 2022. *The medical/health humanities – politics, programs, pedagogies*. New York: Springer.

Jones, T., M. Blackie, R. Garden, and D. Wear. 2017. The almost right word: The move from Medical to Health Humanities. *Academic Medicine* 92:932–935.

Jurecic, A. 2012. *Illness as narrative*. Pittsburgh: Pittsburgh University Press.

Kang, M. C., S. Y. Jung, S. Lee, Y. J. Lee, Y. K. Chung, J. H. Jang, B. Park, and S. Y. Kong. 2025. Causal attributions in patients with breast and gynecological cancers: A scoping review. *Psycho-Oncology* 34:e70253.

Kaplan, R. M. 1990. Behavior as the central outcome in health care. *American Psychologist* 45:1211–1220.

Kaptein, A. A., A. C. Lyons, A. S. Pearson, S. van der Geest, J. Haan, F. Meulenberg, and J. M. Smyth. 2012. Storying stories. *Medical Education Development* 2:24–26.

Kaptein, A. A., J. W. Schoones, P. B. van der Meer, A. Matsuda, M. Murray, L. Heimans, and J. R. Kroep. 2021. Psychosocial determinants of adherence with oral anti- cancer treatment: 'We don't need no education'. *Acta Oncologica* 60:87–95.

Kleinman, A. 1988. *The illness narratives. Suffering, healing, and the human condition*. New York: Basic Books.

Klugman, C. M., and E. G. Lamb, eds. 2019. *Research methods in health humanities*. Oxford: Oxford University Press.

Lawrence, C., T. Mhlaba, K. A. Stewart, R. Moletsane, B. Gaede, and M. Moshabela. 2018. The hidden curricula of medical education: A scoping review. *Academic Medicine* 93:648–656.

Leventhal, H. 2019. Next steps for examining the common-sense of health behaviour. *Health Psychology Review* 13:487–489.

Leventhal, H., L. A. Phillips, and E. Burns. 2016. The Common-Sense Model of Self-Regulation: A dynamic framework for understanding illness self-management. *Journal of Behavioral Medicine* 39:935–946.

O'Mahony, S. 2013. Against narrative medicine. *Perspectives in Biology and Medicine* 56:611–619.

Ousager, J., and H. Johannessen. 2010. Humanities in undergraduate medical education: A literature review. *Academic Medicine* 85:988–998.

Richardson, E. M., N. Schüz, K. Sanderson, J. L. Scott, and B. Schüz. 2017. Illness representations, coping, and illness outcomes in people with cancer: A systematic review and meta-analysis. *Psycho-Oncology* 26:724–737.

Richardson, A. E., E. Broadbent, and R. P. Morton. 2019. A systematic review of psychological interventions for patients with head and neck cancer. *Supportive Care in Cancer* 27:2007–2021.

Rodin, G., E. An, J. Shnall, and C. Malfitano. 2020. Psychological interventions for patients with advanced disease: Implications for oncology and palliative care. *Journal of Clinical Oncology* 38:885–904.
Sain, A. M. de, C. Ruis, M. L. Zomers, M. E. G. ten Hoor-Suykerbuyk, T. Kuunders, F. Y. F. L. de Vos, A. Janssens, and T. Seute. 2025. Towards a definition of an existential approach in cancer patients: A co-produced scoping review. *PLOS One* 20 (9): e0330384.
Skov, M., and M. Nadal. 2025. Can arts-based interventions improve health? A conceptual and methodological critique. *Physics of Life Reviews* 53:239–259.
Sonke J, M. K. B. Tan, J. B. Lee, V. Pesata, A. Akram, T. Golden, et al. 2025. The arts for disease prevention and health promotion: A systematic review. *Nature Medicine* 31:3907–3916.
Strawson, G. 2004. Against narrativity. *Ratio* 17:428–452.
Zhang, Y., X. Chen, R. Li, Y. Wang, Z. Sun, and Q. Li. 2024. Interventions strategies and their efficacy in illness perceptions in patients with cancer: A systematic review and meta-analysis. *European Journal of Oncology Nursing* 70:102599.

2

Reading Cancer

2.1 Depicting Illness

The English modernist writer Virginia Woolf was renowned for her depictions of the human stream of consciousness. True to form, when she herself was bedridden following a nervous breakdown, her thoughts began to flow. She turned to the question of why it was that—at least in her view—writers so seldomly addressed the experience of bodily illness:

> Considering how common illness is, how tremendous the spiritual change that it brings…what wastes and deserts of the soul a slight attack of influenza brings to light…it becomes strange indeed that illness has not taken its place with love and battle and jealousy among the prime themes of literature. (Woolf4 1930, pp. 3–4)

In Woolf's estimation, literary authors were obsessed with matters of the mind but largely ignored the physical experiences of the body. In literature, the body was depicted as little more than "a sheet of plain glass," she suggested, "through which the soul looks straight and clear." However, in retrospect, Woolf's conclusions on this matter may have been overstated.

A. A. Kaptein, B. M. Hughes, *Writing Cancer*,
https://doi.org/10.1007/978-981-95-6501-6_2

Similarly, Susan Sontag, in *Illness as Metaphor*, begins with an equally poignant observation:

> Illness is the night-side of life, a more onerous citizenship. Everyone who is born holds dual citizenship, in the kingdom of the well and in the kingdom of the sick. Although we all prefer to use only the good passport, sooner or later each of us is obliged, at least for a spell, to identify ourselves as citizens of that other place. (Sontag 1978, p. 3)

Were Woolf and Sontag alive today, they might be surprised by the sheer volume of literary works that explore illness—both psychiatric and somatic—and how protagonists and their social contexts navigate these experiences. Numerous academic journals now explore intersections of literature and medicine. Examples include *Art Therapy*, *Hektoen International*, the *International Journal of Art Therapy*, the *Journal of Medical Humanities*, the *Journal of Patient Experience*, *Poetry Therapy*, *Writing Research*, *Medical Humanities*, *Narrative Inquiry*, *Patient Education and Counseling*, *Poetics Today*, and *Psychology of Aesthetics, Creativity, and the Arts*. In addition, a growing body of academic literature addresses these topics (e.g., Bates et al. 2014; Bleakley 2015; Bleakley and Neilson 2022; Crawford et al. 2015; Klugman and Lamb 2019), and academic societies—such as IGEL (the International Society for the Empirical Study of Literature), publisher of *Scientific Study of Literature*—further institutionalise this field.

In other countries too, steps have been taken to develop academic programmes of education and research in the field of health and medical humanities. A wide range of textbooks, journals, and scholarly societies have emerged. In North American colleges, classes in 'Literature and Medicine', 'Medical Humanities', and 'Health Humanities' are increasingly part of medical school curricula. European countries have witnessed similar innovations. Ireland's most prestigious medical school, at Trinity College Dublin, has established a 'Medical and Health Humanities Initiative', aiming to become a world-leading centre for study of the field. The growth of medical humanities has garnered such attention in scholarly circles that a number of historical reviews have now been written (e.g., Bernhardsson 2010; Dalrymple 2021; von Engelhardt 2021a; Hoerni 1994, 2016; Maomai 1997; Schmidt 2018a, b).

2.2 Varieties of Creative Expression

In simple terms, *medical humanities* and *health humanities* are two more or less interchangeable terms used to describe a field of academic research that examines how the creative arts can be deployed to address problems of health and illness.

Medical humanities is often described as an interdisciplinary field that focuses on how the traditional humanities (e.g., literature, philosophy, and history), the social sciences (such as anthropology and cultural studies), and the creative arts (including literature, film, and visual art) can be used in medical education and practice. Virtually any art form can be considered in this way; that said, for present purposes, we will emphasise literature, films, music, and painting.

The scope of medical humanities, in terms of research and clinical application, is wide-ranging, and encompasses literature, film, music, and painting, among many other genres (Kaptein 2021). As ever, it is helpful to make a distinction between the patient and the healthcare provider, as well as to separate 'passive' and 'active' uses of each art form. For example, patients might read novels that are helpful to them (so-called bibliotherapy), or they can produce prose of their own (so-called expressive writing; otherwise—and perhaps more clearly—known as 'experiential writing' or 'self-writing'). Likewise, health professionals too can read novels, in order to deepen their empathy and sensitivity to the experiences of their patients, or, correspondingly, they can write about their clinical experiences. Such activities represent just a small selection of examples; the range of possible activities is as endless as the human potential for creativity (Kaptein et al. 2025).

All these activities have been studied as topics in the field of medical humanities, with most of this research focusing on the use of literature. For example, the benefit of bibliotherapy as an intervention to assist cancer patients has been reviewed in the *Clinical Journal of Oncology Nursing* (Malibiran et al. 2018). Several studies have assessed the use of expressive writing interventions for patients, and have generally found them valuable (Merz et al. 2014; Pennebaker and Evans 2014). The use of humanities classes in medical curricula has also been researched (Ousager and Johannessen 2010). By contrast, the benefits of writing by doctors are not quite so well studied. However, the fact that there are so many examples of this particular genre of literature suggests that, anecdotally at least, many doctors find this activity fulfilling.

While most of the research in medical humanities has centred on the use of literature and creative writing, that is not to say that other art forms have not also been investigated. One group of researchers demonstrated that having patients watch Disney movies during chemotherapy was associated with improvements in emotional functioning and fatigue (Pils et al. 2020). In another study, photography was found to be of marked benefit to cancer patients as a way to help them to describe their daily lives and to express their experiences of distress (Wong et al. 2019), echoing earlier research which had found that women who kept photographic records of their experiences of chemotherapy reported greater feelings of control over their situations (Frith and Harcourt 2007). Several studies have looked at ways to use film in medical education (e.g., Darbyshire and Baker 2012), with the term *cinemeducation* now widely used to describe this approach (e.g., Rueb et al. 2022). Academic books such as *Cinema MD: A History of Medicine on Screen* (Wijdicks 2020) have made it relatively easy to source suitable cinematic material for medical humanities curricula. Films made by doctors themselves may be especially helpful in teaching other physicians about the realities of patients' lives (Rabow et al. 2010).

Many studies have revealed that music interventions can be helpful for alleviating the intensity of emotional, physical, and social suffering in cancer patients (Bradt et al. 2021). For example, music can lessen listeners' feelings of fatigue (Trigueros-Murillo et al. 2023) and of stress (Jeppesen et al. 2019). There has been much less research on whether *playing* music is of benefit to patients, although many high-profile music artists have produced works inspired by, or relating to, cancer, such as David Bowie's *Blackstar* album in 2016, the Belgian singer Jacques Brel's track *Vieillir* from 1977, and the song *Quand c'est?* (which when pronounced in French sounds like 'cancer') by rapper Stromae from 2013.

Researchers have investigated the value of using music in medical education, to help teach students about death and dying (Butler 2009), and in the operating theatre, to help surgeons maintain focus on their work (Fu et al. 2020). It is certainly not unusual for medical schools to provide opportunities to students to participate in music activities: so-called 'medical orchestras' are common around the world (e.g., Subramanian and Brooks 2022; Wong 2012).

Artistic painting has been found to boost quality of life in patients undergoing leukaemia treatment (Mische Lawson et al. 2017). Other research has explored whether asking patients to draw pictures of their own cancers and then comparing them to X-rays can offer useful opportunities to discuss illness with patients (Hoogerwerf et al. 2012). At least for some specialities, medical students appear to learn more from viewing human bodies in artistic paintings than they do from diagrams in medical textbooks (Naghshineh et al. 2008). Many doctors themselves prove to be highly proficient painters; the pioneering British surgeon Roy Calne is one of the most renowned (cf., Calne 1996).

The interface between medicine and the arts has evolved over time. A recent example is the growth of so-called *graphic medicine*, which applies the medium of comics and cartooning to the discourse of healthcare (Williams 2012). Prominent examples of how authors and illustrators have used patients' stories to create comic books and graphic novels include *Cancer Vixen* (Marchetto 2006), *Mom's Cancer* (Fies 2006), and *When David Lost His Voice* (Vanistendael 2012).

2.3 How Cancer Transcends Medicine, Science, and the Humanities

The term *medical humanities* is not to everyone's liking. Many critics consider it to imply an over-emphasis on biomedical concerns, and prefer the term *health humanities* as a way to highlight the broader experiential factors that impinge on a person's well-being (e.g., Jones et al. 2017). (The term *biopsychosocial humanities* has not—heretofore—been coined.)

Correspondingly, much of the published material on these topics have appeared outside the formal 'medical' literature. Medical journals offer important forums for scholarship that are both specialised (e.g., the *Journal of Medical Humanities, Medical Humanities,* and the *Journal of Writing Research*) and generic (e.g., the *Lancet*, the *New England Journal of Medicine*, *JAMA*, and *Annals of Internal Medicine*). But equally pertinent are a number of long-established *non*-medical journals (such as *Art Therapy, Arts & Health,* and the *Journal of Music Therapy*).

In several respects, cancer presents a human experience that transcends medicine, science, and the humanities as a whole, and any evaluation of the field will be required to be expansive rather than narrow. As C. P. Snow (1964) observed in *The Two Cultures,* it can be dangerous to have "two cultures which can't or don't communicate" (p. 98). As we will see in the following chapters, there have been many, many creative attempts to portray the experience of cancer by allowing the multiple cultures involved to learn from—and inspire—each other.

References

Bates, V., A. Bleakley, and S. Goodman, eds. 2014. *Medicine, health and the arts – approaches to the medical humanities*. London: Routledge.

Bernhardsson, K. 2010. *Litterära besvär [Suffering in literature]*. Stockholm: Ellerströms.

Bleakley, A. 2015. *Medical humanities and medical education*. London: Routledge.

Bleakley, A., and S. Neilson. 2022. *Poetry in the clinic – towards a lyrical medicine*. London: Routledge.

Bradt, J., C. Dileo, K. Myers-Coffman, and J. Biondo. 2021. Music interventions for improving psychological and physical outcomes in people with cancer (review). *Cochrane Database of Systematic Reviews* 10 (10): CD006911.

Butler, D. J. 2009. Teaching about the traumatic impact of vehicular crashes: Rock 'n roll never forgets. *Family Medicine* 41:549–551.

Calne, R. 1996. *Art, surgery and transplantation*. London: Williams & Wilkins.

Crawford, P., B. Brown, C. Baker, V. Tischler, and B. Abrams, eds. 2015. *Health humanities*. London: Palgrave.

Dalrymple, T., ed. 2021. *The best medicine – Stories of healing*. New York: A.A. Knopf.

Darbyshire, D., and P. Baker. 2012. A systematic review and thematic analysis of cinema in medical education. *Medical Humanities* 38:28–33.

Fies, B. 2006. *Mom's Cancer*. New York: Abrams.

Frith, H., and D. Harcourt. 2007. Using photographs to capture women's experiences of chemotherapy: Reflecting on the method. *Qualitative Health Research* 17:1340–1350.

Fu, V. X., P. Oomens, V. E. E. Kleinrensink, K. J. Sleurink, W. M. Borst, P. E. Wessels, J. F. Lange, G. J. Kleinrensink, and J. Jeekel. 2020. The effect of preferred music on mental workload and laparoscopic surgical performance in a simulated setting (OPTIMISE): A randomized controlled crossover study. *Surgical Endoscopy* 35:5051–5061.

Hoerni, B. 1994. *Archipel du cancer [Cancer archipelago]*. Paris: La cherche midi éditeur.

Hoerni, B. 2016. Cancer et littérature [Cancer and literature]. *Histoire des Sciences Medicales* 50:199–206.

Hoogerwerf, M. A., M. K. Ninaber, L. N. A. Willems, and A. A. Kaptein. 2012. 'Feelings are facts', Illness perceptions in patients with lung cancer. *Respiratory Medicine* 106:1170–1176.

Jeppesen, E., C. M. Pedersen, K. R. Larsen, E. S. Walsted, A. Rehl, J. Ehrenreich, S. Schnoor, and V. Backer. 2019. Listening to music prior to bronchoscopy reduces anxiety – a randomised controlled trial. *European Clinical Respiratory Journal* 6:1–9.

Jones, T., M. Blackie, R. Garden, and D. Wear. 2017. The almost right word: The move from Medical to Health Humanities. *Academic Medicine* 92:932–935.

Kaptein, A. A. 2021. Writing cancer. *Supportive Care in Cancer* 29:4375–4380.

Kaptein, A. A., W. E. Hanser, J. W. Schoones, P. Boot, J. W. Pennebaker, and B. M. Hughes. 2025. Cancer in poetry – poetry in cancer: A linguistic analysis of poems by poets on their own cancer and on the cancer of their loved ones. *Psycho-Oncology* 34 (10): e70297.

Klugman, C. M., and E. G. Lamb, eds. 2019. *Research methods in health humanities*. Oxford: Oxford University Press.

Malibiran, R., J. D. Tariman, and Amer K. Bibliotherapy. 2018. Appraisal of evidence for patients diagnosed with cancer. *Clinical Journal of Oncology Nursing* 22:377–380.

Maomai, M. 1997. *Krebs schreiben [Writing cancer]*. Mannheim: Röhrig Universitätsverlag.

Marchetto, M. A. 2006. *Cancer Vixen*. New York: Knopfler.

Merz, E. L., R. S. Fox, and V. L. Malcarne. 2014. Expressive writing interventions in cancer patients: A systematic review. *Health Psychology Review* 8:339–361.

Mische, Lawson L., J. Cline, A. French, and N. Ismael. 2017. Patient perceptions of a 1-h art-making experience during blood and marrow transplant treatment. *European Journal of Cancer Care* 26:1–10.

Naghshineh, S., J. P. Hafler, A. R. Miller, M. A. Blanco, S. R. Lipsitz, R. P. Dubroff, S. Khoshbin, and J. T. Katz. 2008. Formal art observation training improves medical students' visual diagnostic skills. *Journal of General Internal Medicine* 2:991–997.

Ousager, J., and H. Johannessen. 2010. Humanities in undergraduate medical education: A literature review. *Academic Medicine* 85:988–998.

Pennebaker, J. W., and J. F. Evans. 2014. *Expressive writing: Words that heal.* Bedford, Indiana: Idyll Arbor.

Pils, S., J. Ott, A. Reinthaller, E. Steiner, S. Springer, and R. Ristl. 2020. Effect of viewing Disney movies during chemotherapy on self-reported quality of life among patients with gynecologic cancer. *JAMA Network Open* 3:1–10.

Rabow, M. W., S. Goodman, S. Chang, M. Berger, and S. Folkman. 2010. Filming the family: A documentary film to educate clinicians about family caregivers of patients with brain tumors. *Journal of Cancer Education* 25:242–246.

Rueb, M., M. Siebeck, E. A. Rehfuess, and L. M. Pfadenhauer. 2022. Cinemeducation in medicine: A mixed methods study on students' motivations and benefits. *BMC Medical Education* 22:172.

Schmidt, N. 2018a. *The wounded self.* Rochester N.Y: Camden House.

Schmidt, N. 2018b. Intertextuality and the transnational in Verena Stefan's Fremdschläfer (2007): Writing breast cancer from beyond the border. In *The wounded self, writing illness in twenty-first-century German literature*, ed. N. Schmidt, 92–113. Rochester NY: Camden House.

Snow, C. P. 1964. *The two cultures.* Cambridge: Cambridge University Press.

Sontag, S. 1978. *Illness as metaphor*. New York: Farrar, Straus Giroux.

Subramanian, R., and M. J. Brooks. 2022. How a medical orchestra cultivates creativity, joy, empathy, and connection. *AMA Journal of Ethics* 24 (7): E584–E589.

Trigueros-Murillo, A., J. Martinez-Calderon, M. J. Casuso-Holgado, P. González-García, and A. M. Heredia-Rizo. 2023. Effects of music-based interventions on cancer-related pain, fatigue, and distress: An overview of systematic reviews. *Supportive Care in Cancer* 31:488.

Vanistendael, J. 2012. *When David Lost His Voice*. London: SelfMadeHero.
von Engelhardt, D. 2021a. Cancer in literature: Between phenomenology and symbolism. In *Ethical challenges in cancer diagnosis and therapy*, ed. A. W. Bauer et al., 275–290. Zurich: Springer Nature Switzerland.
Wijdicks, E. F. M. 2020. *Cinema MD – a history of medicine on screen*. Oxford: Oxford University Press.
Williams, I. C. M. 2012. Graphic medicine: Comics as medical narrative. *Medical Humanities* 38:21–27.
Wong, L. 2012. *Scales to scalpels: Doctors who practice in the healing arts of music and medicine*. New York: Pegasus.
Wong, S. S., T. J. George, M. Godfrey, J. Le, and D. B. Pereira. 2019. Using photography to explore psychological distress in patients with pancreatic cancer and their caregivers: A qualitative study. *Supportive Care in Cancer* 27:321–328.
Woolf, V. 1930. *On being ill*. London: The Hogarth Press.

3

Writing Cancer

This chapter comprises a series of 30 mini-essays, discussing literary works in which cancer is a major theme. We are often humbled by the fine work produced by scholars in the field of literary criticism, and we make no claim to be capable of emulating their insights. Our efforts in *Writing Cancer* are not intended as an exercise in literary criticism per se. Indeed, our project is a little unusual in this respect. On these pages, we are seeking to apply our insights *as psychologists* to what we read in creative literature on cancer, convinced that doings so can help provoke the potential of medical education and medical/health humanities (two domains in which we *do* have considerable experience).

Our selection of works is not presented in any particular order. And it is personal rather than scientific, undoubtedly influenced by our own interests and experiences. Our intention is to present a cross-section of creative paradigms, literary styles, and life experiences that is stimulating for readers. We feel that the texts we have chosen reflect a range of styles and structures, and are both relevant and informative in the context of biopsychosocial cancer care. Works originally written in English, French, German, or Dutch were studied by us in these original languages. For other works, we relied upon published translations.

A. A. Kaptein, B. M. Hughes, *Writing Cancer*,
https://doi.org/10.1007/978-981-95-6501-6_3

3.1 *The Death of Ivan Ilyich*[1]—Leo Tolstoy

Few writers are as renowned as the Russian Count Lev Nikolayevich Tolstoy (1828–1910), better known simply as 'Leo'. Having been nominated for the Nobel Prize for Literature on multiple occasions (and for the Nobel Peace Prize on multiple *other* occasions), Tolstoy is widely regarded as one of the greatest authors ever to have lived. Several of his novels are instantly recognisable as classics, including *War and Peace*, *Anna Kerenina*, and *Resurrection*. Another, *The Death of Ivan Ilyich*, is frequently acclaimed as a masterpiece of literary fiction.

Tolstoy published *The Death of Ivan Ilyich* in 1886. It is a relatively short book—a novella—coming in at around 26,500 words in English (compared to the nearly 600,000 words of *War and Peace*). It tells the story of Ivan Ilyich, a 45-year-old judge, detailing his career, his family, his colleagues, his illness, and, ultimately, his long and painful death. Based on the various symptoms Tolstoy describes, it is clear that Ilyich's demise is the result of pancreatic carcinoma (Bergqvist et al. 2025).

Perhaps unsurprisingly, *The Death of Ivan Ilyich* is frequently recommended to medical students as part of their 'Literature & Medicine' syllabi. The aim is to invite aspiring physicians to immerse themselves in all facets of illness. (Sometimes this does not go as planned. We know of one instance where a group of Finnish medical students got bogged down in technicalities: instead of delving into the meaning of a character's subjective experiences, they became fixated on whether a workable diagnosis could be deduced from the author's text; Lahtinen and Torppa 2007.)

The illness described by Tolstoy proves almost impossible for Ilyich to countenance. His first reaction is to dismiss his many symptoms as simply the effects of a busy professional life. The nagging pain in his side, the taste of iron in his mouth, the increasing fatigue—even the feelings of irritability towards his wife—are all attributed by Ilyich to his ever-hectic schedule, the cut-and-thrust of being a successful judge in a large and demanding district in Russia.

---

[1] For a recent edition, see: Tolstoy, L. (2008). *The Death of Ivan Ilyich and Other Stories*. London: Penguin Classics.

To put it mildly, Ilyich's interactions with medical professionals prove unrewarding for both parties. "It was all just as it was in the law courts," Tolstoy writes, "The doctor put on just the same air towards him as he himself put on towards an accused person." Medical assertiveness is intertwined with clinical equivocation: "The doctor said that so-and-so indicated that there was so-and-so inside the patient, but if the investigation of so-and-so did not confirm this, then he must assume this and that." As the doctors drone on, Ilyich tunes out. According to Tolstoy, he is concerned with only one question: "Was his case serious or not?"

Ilyich's wife and daughter join in the guessing game, while fellow judges squeamishly distance themselves. Ilyich becomes acutely lonely. He concludes that life is just about over, that there is no hope: "his doubts were still unsolved and remained doubts." Only one person unconditionally respects his being ill, the servant Gerasim, who provides care services to Ilyich, washing his buttocks, and allowing Ilyich to rest his feet on his shoulders. Ilyich finds rapport with his butler, and uses the opportunity to recount his life story to Gerasim. Literary scholars often compare Gerasim's role to that of a midwife during childbirth, except here the task is to assist with life's end rather than its beginning. Once again, Picasso's juxtaposition springs to mind: in death, healthcare *charity* is as vital as medical *science*.

Tolstoy's story takes the reader on a personal exploration. The early chapters span years, the later ones just a few days. Initially, the narrative is set in a huge expansive world; by the end of the novel, all there is, is the confinement of a bedroom. A critical turning point is Ilyich's dream about being on a train, in which he no longer knows whether he is riding forwards or backwards. The train is symbolically pulling Ilyich away from the false values of his life: his lustfulness for status, money, and power. With emerging humility, Ilyich achieves an authenticity of experience and acquires a new respect for others. The journey leads to the final phrases of Tolstoy's novel and the end of Ilyich's life: "He drew in a breath, stopped in the midst of a sigh, stretched out, and died."

Tolstoy was a connoisseur of human experience, a true literary psychologist. By describing the way Ilyich's colleagues think about his impending death, he expertly conveys what readers too think about their own mortality. In short, everyone distances themselves from death when it happens to other people. Philosophically, Ilyich realises that his very existence is in question, asking "When I am not, what will there be?" His conclusion is immediate: "There will be nothing." But, by contrast, everyone else in Tolstoy's novel—including the reader—ignores such finality. They—and we—simply carry on living.

In *The Death of Ivan Ilyich*, oncologists can find an abundance of material on the subjectivity of fatal illness. Tolstoy forces us to think about the way the dying view their diseases, but also shows us how their experiences are perceived and discussed (and perhaps dismissed) by those around them. Modern medical research helps to confirm Tolstoy's observations on the complexities—and the importance—of combined communication, and the need to ensure that the diverse voices of patients, caregivers, and doctors are heard and respected. Patient-reported outcomes have been found to be an essential source of data in modern oncology, alongside laboratory test results and additional diagnostics (e.g., Atkinson et al. 2019). Some studies have suggested that allowing patients to tell their stories and participate in the recording of their own symptoms improves their quality of life and may also contribute to improved survival (e.g., Temel et al. 2010). Like Ivan Ilyich, patients value the opportunity to share how they are doing with their doctor. Listening, it appears, pays off.

Tolstoy's depiction of one man's psychological journey to death is profound, compelling, and truly vivid. To some, reading it is as close as humans can get to living through the actual experience involved. "Everyone dies twice," wrote the Brazilian author Dalton Trevisan, "the first time when they read *The Death of Ivan Ilyich*."

3.2 *Patrimony*[2]—Philip Roth

The doctor's first thought is Bell's palsy. The right side of the old man's face no longer belongs to him: the lower eyelid hangs, the cheek is flabby, as though the bone had been hacked away, and the lips stretch diagonally downwards. The old man pushes his flabby cheek with his fingers,

[2] For a recent edition, see: Roth, P. (2008). *Philip Roth: Novels and Other Narratives—The Counterlife, The Facts, Deception, Patrimony*. New York: Library of America.

declaring that he must have been lying on his pillow for too long. His fellow residents—the man is 86 years old and lives in a retirement home—assure him that his paralysis will be gone in a few weeks. Or, at least, that is their experience.

But the paralysis does not go away; in fact, the next thing to happen is that the man becomes deaf in one ear. Eventually, he can only drink through a straw and eat very slowly, in small portions, a clumsy process of one bite followed by another. His ophthalmologist rules out Bell's and his internal medicine specialist requests an MRI. The diagnosis is finally conclusive. The old man has a brain tumour.

A neurosurgeon expresses pessimism and can only observe as the tumour grows over time, pressing further into the man's facial nerve (Romagna et al. 2025). Surgery is proposed and then deferred. A biopsy of the tumour follows. When the old man's son asks the father how he feels, the father answers, "I wish I were dead." The surgeon reports that the tumour has now reached a critical size and that the patient should expect serious problems within a few months.

The old man's son is Philip Roth (1933–2018), the award-winning American novelist and short story writer. He explained the events in a memoir, *Patrimony: A True Story*. As his father declined, the son Roth saw fit to focus on words and to write everything down in prose. He would record his father's decay for posterity, such was "the unseemliness of my profession," as he observed.

Roth describes seeing his father's brain scans and being unable to connect them to the parent he grew up with, a hard-working and frugal man who, over decades, had built a life in the United States for his wife and children. When it was first published in 1991, the cover of *Patrimony* featured a photograph of the father with a four-year-old Philip, along with Philip's brother. The three stand in front of each other, forming a stable pyramid, a symbol of pre-War familial solidity. The image would radiate Calvinism, were it not for the fact that the Roths were descended from a Jewish community in Belarus. Perhaps hardened by life itself, the father Roth was notably stoic. On the day of Philip's mother's funeral, the father began the task of tidying away her clothes while the guests downstairs offered their condolences. "It's better to be concentrated on what has to be done", was his motto, as recorded by Philip in *Patrimony*.

Patrimony presents Philip's recollection of his father's history from the midst of his imminent death, and so is understandably infused with profound reflections on existence. It tells the story of the father's demise in bracing detail. In one scene, the son fishes his father's dentures out of a filthy bathroom, but the mucus and saliva don't trouble him. In another, the father empties his bowels onto the bathroom floor after a painfully long episode of constipation. Philip spends hours cleaning it up. The father makes him swear never to tell anyone about it, a promise that, with ruthless professionalism, Philip felt expired upon his death.

For Philip, the notion of 'patrimony' equates to *heritage* rather than *inheritance*. Money, objects, or family heirlooms, such as sacred prayer rugs or belts, are ultimately valueless. He describes how, when washing his father, he realised that he needed to pay close attention to every experience in order to save his memories carefully. "You mustn't forget anything," he says. Later, when Philip was leaving to return to New York, the father gave him a package wrapped roughly in brown paper bags and marked with the inscription "From a Father to a Son." When Philip opened it, he found his grandfather's 80-year-old shaving mug. Sometimes, family heirlooms can be important memories in their own way.

In a country where the termination of medical treatment can be enmeshed in legal mazes, Philip's father was quick and clear when handling the relevant paperwork. "Send it over and I'll sign," he promised. As with the day of his wife's funeral, there was no point in procrastinating over such chores. Dying is ultimately hard work, and here too, the senior Roth was to prove a diligent labourer.

In the end, in *Patrimony*, Philip shields the reader from his father's actual death. The book is thus more about life, the experience of living with, rather than dying from, a terminal illness. In this account, it is the patient who is the hero, for dying well. There is no talk of heroic medical rescues.

Nonetheless, illness is not a role to be performed alone. Relatives and care providers join in the experience. Caregiving, including that "from a son to a father", can be a truly traumatic task. This is why caregivers, both formal and informal, are deserving of priority in health service budgets (Lambert et al. 2019) and in research (Ruben et al. 2018).

Improving outcomes for family members is an important need in cancer care, albeit an often-overlooked one.

3.3 *Cancer Ward*[3]—Aleksandr Solzhenitsyn

Cancer Ward, by the Russian novelist and dissident Aleksandr Solzhenitsyn (1918–2008), is one of the most renowned works of cancer-related literature. Originally published in Russian in 1966, it appeared in English in 1968. Framed as a semi-autobiographical novel, the book leads the reader into the cancer ward of a small and squalid hospital in Tashkent, Uzbekistan, a year after the death of Joseph Stalin. Stalin's death and its aftermath were traumatic for Russian society, and Solzhenitsyn's cancer novel is infused with recurring political symbolism.

Solzhenitsyn allows every character to shine in the spotlight, be they patients, doctors, nurses, relatives, or visitors. While some have benefitted from Stalinism, others have lost out, with the ever-present impending threat of mortality serving to accentuate each character's struggles with their resulting moral responsibilities. The novel shows how cancer raises the ethical stakes, whether a person lives with cancer, works with it, survives it, or dies from it. One character, an unfortunate radiologist, spends so many hours providing care to patients that she herself is eventually made ill by radiation exposure, cruelly struck down by her own dedication, and ending up with cancer herself.

Like Solzhenitsyn himself, the main character, a cancer patient called Oleg Kostoglotov, is a former soldier and political prisoner, currently in exile. Kostoglotov frequently blends reflections on illness with questions about the health of Russia, employing the novel's key symbolism of cancer to describe the prevailing political situation. Memorably, he asks: "A man dies from a tumour, so how can a country survive with growths like labour camps and exiles?" He eventually concludes that Russia's decline is terminal and that any apparent periods of remission are sadly illusory. (Nonetheless, it is notable that Solzhenitsyn has Oleg survive his illness and leave the cancer ward alive at the end of the novel.)

Ironically, it was common in Russia at that time to use military imagery when discussing physical illness. Patients were frequently described as "battling" a "hostile" disease that had "invaded" their bodies. Even cancer cells were spoken of as a type of "landing craft", vividly embellishing the

[3] For a recent edition, see: Solzhenitsyn, A. (2003). *Cancer Ward.* London: Vintage.

metaphor of military infiltration (Kaptein and Lyons 2010). As such, in having Oleg depict the country's demise as resonating with terminal cancer, Solzhenitsyn rounds out the allegory in an especially effective manner.

The events of *Cancer Ward* span a relatively short period of time, following the fates of its protagonists for about two months. There are a variety of archetypal patients: some who are in denial of the reality of illness, others who seek miracle cures from alternative medicine, some who are silent and cantankerous, and, strikingly, a girl, about to undergo a mastectomy, who asks a boy to kiss her breast ("Today it was a marvel," Solzhenitsyn writes, "Tomorrow it would be in the bin"). The staff too are recognisable: the petulant surgeon ("Well what have we here? Another nice little cancer!"), the empathetic oncologist, who allows her patients to see their X-rays, and, of course, the altruistic radiologist who denies her own symptoms. Nurses bring books on pathological anatomy to patients who want to know more than their doctors are telling them. One nurse invites a patient home to have sex for the last time. Visitors too try to entice patients to leave the cancer ward and go home. Cancer is uncontainable. It will not let itself be walled in.

Solzhenitsyn's intertwining narratives highlight how many dimensions of illnesses are pertinent only to those who have them. Often an illness as viewed by a patient will look quite different to that perceived by a doctor, who will focus on the physical. Psychologists sometimes try to delineate these various aspects by classifying so-called illness perceptions, usually by distinguishing perceptions that relate to *identity*, *causes*, *consequences*, *timeline*, *influence*, *understanding*, and *emotions*.

Perceptions of *identity* relate to the labels and metaphors that patients apply to their own illness, which are often more influential than reality in determining a patient's actions. For example, in one exchange, Solzhenitsyn describes how a patient with a large neck tumour sees nothing wrong with their body ("I have cancer of nothing," he insists, "I have no cancer whatsoever"). Solzhenitsyn illustrates the diverse *causes* that patients typically perceive, often favouring psychosomatic attributions ("the moment he loses heart, there's too much potassium, and you might as well order the coffin"). The *consequences* of an illness are often perceived as all-encompassing ("Her world had capsized, the entire arrangement of her existence was disrupted"). Separately, its *timeline* can feel particularly daunting, especially where cancer is expected to be terminal ("The question is now, how to postpone it, and how much time do I stand to gain—months or years?"). Perceptions of *treatment* are obviously important, but often in ways that deviate from medical orthodoxy ("Extra treatment means extra torment. There'll be radiation sickness, vomiting…what's the point?"), resulting in a focus on perceived *influence* over the disease. Another important illness perception relates to the degree of *understanding* that a patient wishes to acquire ("I must have a look at it and try and work things out. For myself")—or not ("You decide whether I'm to go into hospital or not and I'll go, but I don't want to know the details"). And of all illness perceptions, perhaps those relating to *emotions* can be most overwhelming ("Within a few hours, that first evening in the ward, Pavel Nikolayevich became haunted with fear…you felt the door to all your past life had been slammed behind you, and the life here was so vile that it frightened you more than the actual tumour."; Liu et al. 2025).

Solzhenitsyn himself was a patient at that cancer ward in Tashkent, and wrote his novel on handwritten sheets of paper that were smuggled out of the hospital by friends. Previously, he had spent eight years in a prison camp after the Second World War. The way his novel implied parallels between Russian politics and cancer invited more political persecution, and Solzhenitsyn was exiled from the Union of Soviet Writers after *Cancer Ward* was published in the United Kingdom. Solzhenitsyn was awarded the Nobel Prize for literature in 1970 but continued to draw criticism from the communist regime. He was eventually deported from the Soviet Union in 1974, but returned to Russia in the 1990s after the regime had collapsed.

3.4 *When Breath Becomes Air*[4]—Paul Kalanithi

Every doctor does it: search through the electronic patient file for information about themselves. However, few go through what Paul Kalanithi (1977–2015) experiences when viewing his own MRI scan on the

[4] For a recent edition, see: Kalanithi, P. (2016). *When Breath Becomes Air*. New York: Random House.

computer screen. Kalanithi, a neurosurgical trainee at Stanford University, had undergone testing after developing a set of symptoms that, singly, would merely have been odd, but, in combination, seemed to be worrying: unexplained weight loss, a new pain in his back, pressure on his chest, night sweats, a niggling cough. An early X-ray had shown little awry, leading his doctor to surmise that he was suffering from work-related stress. But when his symptoms deteriorated, an MRI was ordered. Viewing the image on the screen, Paul's gravest suspicions are now confirmed. Both his lungs are full of shadows, there is a lobe with lumps in his liver, and his spinal column appears distorted. Thirty-six years old and on track for a professorship—Yale, Stanford, and Harvard had already sent him job offers—Paul now knows that his life will likely be foreshortened. Accordingly, he directs his academic effort to the task of recording his experiences in writing. *When Breath Becomes Air,* the bestselling book he produces, would eventually be published posthumously, in 2016, the year after its author has died.

When Breath Becomes Air traces Paul's experience of what was going on in his own body. At first, he attributes his ailments to overwork, sleep loss, and careless eating. It is Lucy, his wife, herself a specialist in internal medicine, who insists he make an appointment with a doctor. The doctor appears to have some difficulty dealing with a medically trained patient such as Paul. When Paul tells her that he thinks he might have isthmic spondylolisthesis, she has to search for the term on Google. When he wishes to discuss Kaplan-Meier curves with her, she refuses. She tells him that he must accept her as his attending physician. Paul, dressed in a patient gown, is reluctant to discard his medical identity (Orr et al. 2025).

Figuratively speaking, Paul's medical white coat bore heavily on his shoulders. "That identity as a physician – my identity – no longer mattered," he writes when describing his sense of powerlessness in the face of physical disease. In his mind, being struck down by cancer was nothing to romanticise, but was a form of ruination: "Severe illness wasn't life-altering, it was life-shattering. It felt less like an epiphany – a piercing burst of light, illuminating What Really Matters – and more like someone had just firebombed the path forward." After his first round of chemotherapy, he sees from his own CT scan that his cancer appears to be in remission. But after resuming work, having revelled in discovering that he still had all his surgical skills, he suddenly faints while performing an operation. He must discard his surgical scrubs once more, and resume his role as a patient.

A few days later, a new MRI shows a picture that is even more serious than before. Paul is soon overwhelmed by new, crueler symptoms: "Eating, normally a source of great pleasure, was like drinking seawater. Suddenly, all of my joys were salted." He is seen by a plethora of doctors. Unlike other cancer patients, Paul's advanced medical knowledge enables him to taxonomise this "pantheon of specialists" with individual precision, all the "medical intensivists, nephrologists, gastroenterologists, endocrinologists, infectious disease specialists, neurosurgeons, general oncologists, thoracic oncologists, otolaryngologists." Even while "floating through varying levels of consciousness," he sees and recognises them all.

Due to wounds on his fingertips (as a consequence of neuropathy), Paul wears woollen gloves while typing. Eventually he is no longer able to complete his book. After he dies, in the same hospital he worked in, his wife carries on the writing and finishes the manuscript.

Paul's great difficulty in playing the patient role reflected his sheer dedication to professionalism and career. This relentlessness to endeavour was lifelong. Even as a child, he applied himself meticulously. His parents fostered his agility, forcing him to eat with his left hand so as to help him become ambidextrous. During his pre-medical school years, he studied English literature, further refining his rounded sense of the human experience. Later, when recalling his medical training in the early chapters of *When Breath Becomes Air*, he displays a thoughtfulness about life and death that had long been core to his medical philosophy. He recalls the way his anatomy teachers insisted that students refer to the cadavers they were dissecting as "donors," seeing this as a humanising measure designed to diminish the risk of "your grandparents being hacked to pieces by wisecracking twenty-two-year-old medical students." Later, when he begins to see patients, he is struck by their endless individuality. He cannot help but develop emotional attachments with them. Dutifully, and with touching detail, he lists some of "the people I saw die" in his first year as a doctor. This acknowledgement of mortality serves to foreshadow his own later death (Philipp et al. 2019).

The cover of *When Breath Becomes Air* depicts a single blue feather, a metaphor for the lightness of respiration, a symbol of how what leaves the lungs infuses (and thus is part of) the wider atmosphere. In the same way, doctors are part of a wider human ecology, and so themselves are joined to their patients. Kalanithi argues that the doctorish habit of seeing people's bodies as machines—brought in for repair like engines to a mechanic—might help protect physicians from the suffering caused by empathy. However, it comes at a cost to those who are ill. "How little do doctors understand the hells through which we put patients," he writes.

For Kalanithi, medical practice requires not just biological expertise, but the ability to connect on a human level. Perhaps revealing his early studies of literature (Kaptein and Thong 2018), he emphasises how important it is for doctors to carefully consider language, narrative, and framing when sharing their feedback. The impressions left by doctors on their patients can forever colour how a family views their loved one's eventual death. "When there's no place for the scalpel," he writes, "words are the surgeon's only tool."

3.5 *The Death of a Beekeeper*[5]—Lars Gustafsson

In many European countries, there is a tradition of "telling the bees" about important events in their beekeepers' lives. When the British Queen Elizabeth II died in 2022, this task was handed to the Royal Beekeeper, whose official duty was to inform the bees at Buckingham Palace that the old monarch had passed away and a new king had ascended to the throne. He was required to make the announcement multiple times, once at each hive, having first knocked on the hive's door to get the bees' attention.

Tradition dictates that if bees are not told of their keeper's death, they may abandon the hive, become infertile, or stop producing honey. In *The Death of a Beekeeper*, a 1978 novel by the Swedish writer Lars Gustafsson

[5] For a recent edition, see: Gustafsson, L. (1981). *The Death of a Beekeeper*. New York: New Directions.

(1936–2016), the lead character Lars Lennart Westin, an unemployed divorcee who keeps bees and lives alone with his dog, deliberately decides to challenge this practice. In so doing, he seeks to take control of his own illness—and therefore of his own *destiny*—by framing his own personal experiential narrative (Bondevik et al. 2016).

Aged just 40, Westin receives a letter from the hospital containing the results of his diagnostic examination. He decides not to know what the doctors had found: casually, he uses the unopened envelope to light a fire in the hearth. "Either the letter says that it's nothing bad," he muses, "Or it says that I have cancer and am going to die…The smartest thing for me would be not to open it, because if I don't open it, there is still going to be some kind of hope." Westin understands that any latitude offered by hope will be unable to make his physical pain disappear. However, he concludes that a pain for which he does not know the cause will be more bearable than one produced by an identified, named illness. A "general pain" is something he can integrate into his life. "Why shouldn't I be able to do that?" he wonders.

Westin lives in a wooden house in central Sweden, where he struggles with the cold winter and the pain that infuses throughout his body. Even though modern medicine has produced many ways to manage pain very effectively, Westin sacrifices the opportunity to avail of these treatments in order to avoid being informed of the underlying diagnosis. He wishes to deal with his pain on his own, regardless of the consequences. As a divorcee who lives alone, perhaps his priorities are just different. He feels that he can decide what his own reality will entail.

Gustafsson's novel vividly portrays the limits of this philosophy. To the reader, the trajectory is clear from the beginning; metastatic spleen cancer is mentioned on the very first page. Even Westin's dog is aware that something is wrong, piercing the illusion by literally smelling trouble and avoiding its owner "as if I stink" (a remarkable observation for the 1970s, in pre-empting later technologies that would allow cancer doctors to analyse exhaled breath samples using electronic e-nose systems; e.g., Binson et al. 2021). Westin persists with his plan, instead taking his dog outside, for long walks along the peninsula where he lives.

Westin develops a number of mental strategies to manage his pain. He hangs his pain on a tree he walks past. He sticks his pain to a fence. He throws his pain into the lake. He is committed to being in control of his suffering, telling himself that pain is only painful when it hurts ("It must be paradise if the pain has stopped. That means we live in paradise as long as we are not in pain"). He views pain as an animate entity, something that comes and goes of its own accord, as if it had a mind of its own. "That gives me comfort too," he explains, "like when a lonely person finds comfort in a pet." But as time passes, he finds pain to be an unsentimental companion. Pain tolerates no rivalry. "The pain is no longer a pet," he complains, "it is a hideous white-hot force taking over my nervous system, exploding in every nerve."

Unable to entirely reframe his situation, Westin is nagged by intrusive thoughts about the potential reality of his illness. After his pain briefly subsides, he resolves to wait at least a week before allowing himself to hope it has gone forever. When it returns, he is tormented by its meaning. He formulates a manic rationalisation: "Since I burned that letter, the hospital hasn't said anything. If it really was cancer, then they would have contacted me again. So: it was nothing, some kind of inflammation." Unfortunately, however, even this is insufficient: "But what if they misplaced the papers?" he ends up asking himself. Reverting once again to self-protection, he realises that he is avoiding the letterbox (Łuczyk et al. 2024).

Further distraction is provided when two schoolboys call by, asking Westin about his secluded life in his strange wooden house. He tells them stories about dragons and aliens. The boys help to bring him back to earth, forcing him to reconnect with the reality of his own life story, to reflect on all those past experiences of relationships and infatuation, of sex and of sun. Briefly, the boys' own zest for life helps to reinforce Westin's resilience in the face of pain. But ultimately the pain can no longer be controlled. "I knew it had only been a hiatus," he concedes, "the unpleasant resemblance between pain and pleasure. Both demand total attention, everything else falls away…" Despite all of his commitment, Westin's coping strategies are ultimately insufficient (Porter et al. 2019).

While many writers have written about physical pain, pain as specific to cancer is described relatively rarely. Gustafsson's *The Death of a Beekeeper* is therefore especially valuable. It makes clear that pain can be an overwhelming aspect of cancer, and yet can make a patient live their life with more intensity. It also showcases the way in which people can rationally construct their own life narratives in order to offset the physical—and mental—torture of pain, at least temporarily.

On the final page of the novel, an ambulance drives down a snow-covered road towards the hospital. Whether the bees have been informed of the fate of their keeper, the author is unsure.

3.6 *Mars*[6]—Fritz Zorn

"My family is quite degenerate and I suspect that I myself am also genetically predisposed and affected by my environment. Of course I also have cancer, which naturally follows from the aforementioned." So reads the opening statements of *Mars*, an autobiographical book by the Swiss author Fritz Zorn (1944–1976). 'Zorn'—the German word for 'anger'—was the author's chosen *nom de plume*. His real surname was Angst—the German word for 'fear'.

It is perhaps not merely ironic that the author's names were infused with negative emotion. In many ways, the same could be said of the entirety of *Mars* itself. The book is an extended diatribe against the world in general, in which the author complains about his surroundings, his friends, his upbringing (despite having been raised in an extremely privileged and wealthy Zürich suburb), and his sex life. As Zorn has never been able to attract a girlfriend, many critics identify *Mars* as a pioneering work of 'incel' literature.

It is Zorn's belief that his propensity to negative emotions has led him to develop cancer. This notion—that cancer might sometimes be caused by psychological degradation, such as that resulting from personal (or familial) failings, emotional turmoils, or mental stress—is a longstanding belief in human culture. Nowadays we are aware that it is tendentious. While biomedical science can trace clear causal links between mental states and, say, disease-relevant cardiovascular function, claims that stress

[6] For a recent English-language edition, see: Zorn, F. (1982). *Mars*. New York: Alfred A. Knopf.

can precipitate the onset of *cancer* (as opposed to its progression) lack as convincing an empirical evidence base.

Nonetheless, Zorn is convinced that his cancer is psychosomatic. He cites, as his authority, the Austrian psychoanalyst Wilhelm Reich, whose 1940s ideas about illness have, in more recent decades, been discarded as pseudoscience. Zorn's view is that his cancer cells have resulted from suppressed emotions and misunderstood sexual impulses. He blames his illness on "*verschluckte Tränen*", or literally, on his "swallowed tears".

"It was as if all the tears that I hadn't cried and hadn't wanted to cry in my life had collected in my neck," he writes, "and had formed this tumour there, because they had not been able to reach their proper destiny, which is to be cried…" In Zorn's view, cancer is therefore a "disease of the soul." Notwithstanding today's biomedical science literature, popular beliefs in the power of the human mind to afflict a person with cancer continue to be widely held.

But it is not just the general public who have been seduced by such a notion. Many scientists have pursued the idea with research, and some have extended the logic by making grand claims to the effect that psychological therapies can be used, as antidotes, to *cure* these psychologically induced cancers. Some of these researchers have touted the idea of a 'Type C' or 'cancer prone' personality, a cluster of characteristics that—allegedly—predisposes certain people to cancer risk. The problem is that many of these findings have been impossible to replicate, and some of the studies are so suspicious as to have attracted accusations of fraud (Pelosi 2019).

The problem with psychosomatic attributions is that patients who truly believe them may be disinclined to engage in treatments they feel are 'too biomedical'. Why trust the oncologist, they can ask themselves, when the oncologist doesn't truly understand *my* cancer? When a physician criticises their patient's psychosomatic beliefs, there is a high risk that the patient will feel alienated. The resulting loss of the 'buy-in' serves to degrade the doctor-patient relationship and reduce the likelihood of a successful medical outcome, by undermining the patient's motivation to follow the doctor's advice. Physicians who want to avoid this problem must hold back on their scientific criticisms.

Some research has suggested that it is possible to work with patients in ways that indirectly enhance, or even change, their cancer beliefs. Interventions aimed at building coping and self-management skills while improving awareness of cancer biology have been somewhat successful in improving quality of life, and in some cases treatment outcomes (Richardson et al. 2019). Many expressive writing interventions are based on these themes (Merz et al. 2014).

In the 1970s, the young Fritz Angst felt he needed to change his name when writing a book about himself, in order to protect his family. It is unclear whether such sensitivity would be required in today's age of oversharing and confessionalism. Zorn's idea that cancer is caused by suppressed tears may also be dated, but the belief that human minds are somewhat involved in carcinogenesis has certainly endured. Implicit in Zorn's analysis is an endorsement of the 'just world' hypothesis, a philosophical bias that makes us believe that, in the end, everyone gets what they deserve. Psychosomatic theories about cancer-prone personalities are essentially theories of karma.

It is striking that, of all the things Zorn complains about in *Mars*, having cancer is not really one of them. Such is his nihilism towards the world that, to Zorn, cancer comes almost as a relief. He welcomes it, as it confirms his prior beliefs about the consequences of his psychological experiences. He would not have expected anything else (Fang et al. 2025).

It was on the day before Zorn died of a lymphoma, at the age of 32, that a publisher decided to publish his manuscript as a book. Zorn was unconscious by then. The final sentence he wrote was: "I declare myself in a state of total war." His anger, if not his fear, outlived him.

3.7 *The Black Swan*[7]—Thomas Mann

The prolific German novelist Thomas Mann (1875–1955) was awarded the Nobel Prize for Literature in 1929, but continued to produce acclaimed work for another quarter of a century, writing his last completed work of fiction in the 1950s at the age of 78. This was the novella

[7] For a recent edition, see: Mann, T. (1990). *The Black Swan*. Berkeley: University of California Press.

Die Betrogene, or 'The Deceived One', published in English as *The Black Swan*.

The story centres around a 50-year-old widow, Rosalie von Tümmler, who suffers headaches, nervousness, and amenorrhea, and believes she is entering the menopause. Mann surrounds Rosalie with three main characters: her daughter Anna, who is chaste, her quiet son Eduard, who is almost invisible, and Eduard's American tutor Ken, who comes to occupy most of her attention. While Anna becomes concerned at her mother's weary eyes and yellowish skin, it is Ken's white teeth, broad shoulders, muscular arms, and American accent that fascinate Rosalie (and indeed her friends).

Rosalie's interest in Ken develops into infatuation. Her emerging sexual awareness sees her become newly re-invigorated. Not only does her sex drive return, but so also does her menstrual cycle. This she describes to Anna as a "victory" and a "miracle", a true source of elation. "It has come back, after such a long hiatus," she declares, "all natural, as befits a mature, vivacious woman!"

Rosalie and Ken soon become entangled. A boat trip on the Rhine takes them to a castle with a moat, where black swans keep a watchful eye on visitors. When Rosalie tries to feed the swans some bread—bread that Ken had kept warm with his body—things start to go wrong. Flexing its mighty neck and fiery red beak, one particularly aggressive swan coming dangerously close to Rosalie, startling her. "Did you see him hissing at me?!" she cries. Freud couldn't have put it better.

Rosalie and Ken, sexually enthralled with each other, plan to meet in her bedroom the next evening. But early that day, Rosalie is found bleeding and unconscious in her bed. The symbolism intended by the appearance of the black swan—and its red beak—becomes ominously apparent. Rosalie is hospitalised with presumed ovarian cancer (Nogueria et al. 2025). Gravely, and with no little trepidation, an oncologist announces: "*ut aliquid fieri videatur*"—which roughly translates as "we must be *seen* to be doing something!" (von Grueningen et al. 2018). He performs an incision on her abdomen in order to examine her organs, and then attempts some drastic surgery, until it becomes obvious that any treatment will be futile. In the end, nature is merciful. Rosalie dies "a gentle death", Mann writes, "regretted by all who knew her."

Mann consulted a number of medical specialists before writing *The Black Swan*, carefully familiarising himself with the clinical picture, diagnosis, and surgical treatments for cancer. His description of Rosalie's medical examination employs unusually accurate technical language. That being said, Mann focuses on the story to be told rather than providing endless medical detail, and some oncologists now debate whether Rosalie might have suffered from cervical rather than ovarian cancer (Dietl 2004).

Mann's own experiences also came into play. His story of Rosalie's illness was influenced by an anecdote that his wife Katia used to tell him. In addition, and crucially, Mann had himself survived cancer, having undergone bold invasive surgery to remove a carcinoma from his lung in 1946. The procedure was conducted by the American surgeon William Adams in Chicago. Its operative complexity—and the fame of the patient—were such that the operation is regarded by many modern surgeons as being especially significant to the history of medicine (Naef and William 1998). Its success kept Mann alive for the next nine years (after which the novelist would die from an unrelated cardiovascular illness).

The Black Swan, while short, is a multi-layered novel. It incorporates many themes that recur throughout Mann's writing, such as the entangling of love, illness, and death. The character of Ken is modelled after beautiful American boys that Mann had found attractive in his own life, a theme he famously explored in his earlier masterpiece, *Death in Venice*. *The Black Swan* also deals with how many people resort to denial as a way to cope with fear. Mann himself relied heavily on this form of coping, as was typical for many gay men during the early twentieth century. Mann's sexuality was central to his fiction-writing, but was only ever explicitly expressed in his personal (and private) diaries.

The Black Swan is often presented to medical trainees as part of their education on doctor-patient communication. Teachers use the novel to discuss with students the themes of denial, grief, symptom perception, and illness behaviour. Educators who have done this have found that students often focus on the role of oestrogen in contributing to ovarian carcinoma (Lahtinen and Torppa 2007), an illustration of how for doctors, the medical/technical often ends up distracting from the emotional/experiential. It can also be noted that Mann's novel is somewhat restricted by the author's own positionality, as a story about menstruation that is written by a man. As such, in education, the book may offer a useful way to stimulate important discussions about gender representation in medicine.

Mann died in 1955, aged 80, himself experiencing a gentle death similar to the one he chose for Rosalie. "We also wish for ourselves to die like this," he had written. *Die Betrogene* would ultimately be his final work: truly, his swan song.

3.8 *Cancer Vixen*[8]—Marisa Acocella Marchetto

To some literary aficionados, graphic novels are not really novels at all, but overblown comic books. However, anyone who doubts the ability of graphic novelists to produce stirring works of existential fiction, or to address profound and challenging themes and social issues, should perhaps familiarise themselves with 'graphic medicine' (Green and Myers 2010). This is the field that uses graphic narratives to convey medical pathographies to a diverse range of patients, and indeed to doctors.

Graphic novels might be seen as a modern form of literature, but they have evolved over more than a century and across many different cultures (Sabin 1996). Part of their appeal—and much of their richness—arises from the multimodal ways in which authors are liberated to give effect to their creative visions. Images are employed not merely as 'pictures' in the diagrammatic sense of the term, but also as tools with which metaphors and allegories can be developed. The skills of a graphic novelist are therefore akin to those of a cinematographer, while also incorporating the traditional wordsmithing that typifies the classical novelist.

Revered medical journals such as the *BMJ*, *JAMA*, and the *Journal of Clinical Oncology* have each published examples of graphic medicine. The flagship Canadian journal *CMAJ* proactively invites authors to submit graphic medicine manuscripts. There are now learned societies devoted to

[8] For a recent edition, see: Marchetto, M. A. (2006). *Cancer Vixen: A True Story*. New York: Alfred A. Knopf.

the study of graphic medicine, along with conferences, symposia, and other scholarly events. Many medical databases link to dedicated journals, such as the *Journal of Graphic Novels and Comics*. Websites such as *www.graphicmedicine.org* and *www.mednarratives.com* provide physicians and researchers with endless materials to help show patients how people live with their conditions. When patients are shown a vivid story in an easily accessible medium, the consoling message is clear: "You are not alone" (Williams 2012).

Cancer Vixen, by Marisa Acocella Marchetto (1962–), is perhaps one of the most famous examples of the genre. Its cover is powerful in conveying its core message: this author—who was diagnosed with cancer three weeks before her wedding day but still went ahead with the ceremony—does not consider herself a cancer 'victim'. She is vibrant, astute, and desirable. She can be seen literally kicking cancer out of this world. She, the cover shows us, is a cancer *vixen.*

Marchetto's story is autobiographical and will be familiar to most medical oncologists. But for non-medical readers, its enduring realities are striking. The author experiences what countless people with cancer go through: invasive diagnostic procedures and therapeutic measures that have grave psychosocial consequences.

The book starts with a bittersweet telling of the author's life in New York., B.C. ("before cancer"), where life's greatest stressors include such wedding-preparation minutiae as what shoes might be preferred for the big day. And then cancer strikes. "Cancer your wedding!" the author's wordplay barks at her. "Cancer your career! Cancer your life!"

Marchetto depicts her story with brutal and disconcerting images, wild colours, and often-aggressive calligraphy. Showing her having dinner with her partner, wine glasses on the table suggest a classic romantic mood, but this is offset by what appears on the blood-red wall behind the couple: the word 'cancer', written repeatedly, hundreds of times.

And yet, the book is also crafted in ways that make the reader (or viewer?) laugh. In a mammography scene, Marchetto graphically illustrates the shape a woman's breast takes when placed under the device. This gets her thinking. She wonders aloud: "Why don't they examine testes like this?"

In another scene, a woman who learns about the writer's potentially life-limiting illness concludes that Marchetto's handsome fiancé will soon be single again. Even though Marchetto *is standing right in front of her*, the woman takes the opportunity to make her move. "*I'm* not sick," she breezily points out, happy to try to seduce the man as if Marchetto was no longer even present. "Call me!"

Set in the United States, some of the themes in *Cancer Vixen* reflect the particular perils of that country's healthcare system. One significant source of stress is the fact that Marchetto has allowed her health insurance to lapse, adding grave financial implications to her illness. Disaster is avoided when it is discovered that her (now) husband's medical insurance can cover some of her treatment.

When it comes to physical disease, most people are visual thinkers; they imagine their bodies as visual forms. It is for this reason that nowadays, during medical consultations, doctors often find that drawing pictures helps them to explain their point. They draw pictures of the organs, the location of the pathology, and even the treatment options. Marchetto's compelling disease narrative typifies the power of graphic medicine to effectively encapsulate a patient's point of view.

It is as useful for patients to draw as it is for doctors. Patients' visual depictions of ill-health—for example, in the form of daggers, tears, and lightning bolts (Broadbent et al. 2019)—vividly exhibit the distinction between 'disease' (the biological state) and 'illness' (the experience). Moreover, when patients are invited to sketch anatomical diagrams of their bodies, their drawings can provide useful insights about their experiences of treatment that are far more informative than answers provided using questionnaires (Lo-Fo-Wong et al. 2014).

In the end, the *Cancer Vixen* triumphs over her illness. And in real life too, Marchetto continues to prosper. Successful chemotherapy was followed by beneficial radiotherapy, and there is now talk of *Cancer Vixen* being made into a movie (Nisiraiou et al. 2025).

A portion of royalties from each sale of the book is donated to breast cancer research. In 2006, a year after she finished treatment, Marchetto established a charitable foundation, The Cancer Vixen Fund. The fund is dedicated to helping other patients become cancer vixens too, providing state-of-the-art mammograms to uninsured women in New York—for free.

3.9 *Wit*[9]—Margaret Edson

The book is only 80 pages long. Author Margaret Edson (1961–) does not need much space to highlight her drama, set in a patient room in a university medical centre. The protagonist, 50-year-old Vivian, pushes an IV pole with a venous catheter attached while wearing two patient gowns, one with the bow on the stomach, the other with the bow on the back. Such details reflect the writer's own extensive experience as a nurse in American oncology departments (van Duin and Kaptein 2013). Edson's 1995 play, *Wit*—sometimes stylised as *W;t*—won a Pulitzer Prize for Drama, and has since become acclaimed as a landmark in medical theatre (Greer et al. 2018). A 2001 film adaptation featured the Hollywood legend Emma Thompson in its lead role; a 2012 production on Broadway gave the part to Cynthia Nixon, of *Sex and the City* fame.

Wit starts with Vivian literally welcoming the audience, nodding and waving to them, asking how things are going. Vivian is a university English professor—Edson herself was for a time a teacher of English—and the play deftly experiments with form while exploring the consoling implications of literature and language. The 'wit' of the play's title refers to a quality of the poetry of John Donne, which Vivian recites as a means of rehearsing her thoughts, and her feelings, about illness. "Death Be Not Proud", one of the most famous of Donne's sonnets, proves especially useful in this regard.

Vivian clearly does not want to be a patient, and prefers asking other people how *they* are feeling. She maintains this coping strategy as much as she can (von Grueningen et al. 2018). When the doctors come by, with their interrogations and briefings, she is unable to avoid the issue of her own state of health. But as a professor of English, Vivian can't help but become enthralled by the words she hears when her attending physician describes stage four ovarian cancer. For her, medical terms like 'insidious', 'destructive', or 'invasive' are loaded with literary allusions and are each worthy of a seminar. Their precise medical meanings are gradually lost as she ponders their thematic resonance.

[9] For a recent edition, see: Edson, M. (1999). *W;t*. London: Faber and Faber.

Vivian constantly struggles to locate herself as the object of other people's endeavours. After she gives her name to a technician, the technician asks "Doctor?", wanting to know what physician had ordered the test. Vivian hears the question but misinterprets it. "Yes," she replies, "I have a PhD."

Later, Dr Posner, an oncology research fellow, comes by to examine Vivian. Before he begins, he tells her that he has attended her lectures on English literature. "You can't get into medical school unless you're well-rounded," he explains. Vivian is somewhat cautious about this versatility and is not convinced that her former student has mastered the importance of language. After four short questions ("How old are you? Are you married? Are your parents living? How and when did they die?"), he summarily declares, "Well, that about does it for your life history." Vivian is taken aback. Is that really all there is to her "life history"?

After experiencing the standard hospital ritual of 'Grand Rounds'—where, as a means of medical education, a senior doctor brings a small group of juniors and students, from bed to bed, to serve as an audience while they treat their patients on the ward—Vivian, for one, does not find the affair to be particularly laden with grandeur. Ever attentive to the details of discourse, in her mind the doctor's utterances are just not that educational. Instead of getting to the point, the senior doctor prefers to skirt around the main issue. Vivian recalls how once she was a teacher, reducing complexity into discrete pieces that her students could digest. Now, she realises, she herself is just subject matter, a lesson to be taught.

The power of language can be as much in its tone as in its content. When Vivian is transferred to an isolation ward, the department head unconvincingly tries to pass it off as no big deal: "Isolation is no problem. Couple of days. Think of it as a vacation." The contrast between how doctors abuse language while professors obsess over it is stark.

It is as though Vivian's doctors not only fail to see the point of communication as a concept, they almost hold the idea with contempt. Posner explains to Vivian that he was trained in doctor–patient communication, but only because it was obligatory. In reality, he just doesn't care about stuff like that. "There's a whole course on bedside manners in med school," he recalls. "It's required. Colossal waste of time for researchers…

Like we have to hold hands to discuss creatinine clearance. Just cut the crap, I say" (Lefkovits et al. 2024).

In the end, it is Nurse Susie who succeeds in reassuring Vivian in an authentic way. Tellingly, she breaks the ice not with words, but by sharing a popsicle with her patient. Susie's warmth is communicated to Vivian's satisfaction. This enables Vivian to finally focus on her cancer, and to make important decisions that had previously been avoided through self-distraction. Vivian exercises her choice to avail of a 'Do Not Resuscitate' (DNR) order, indicating that she wants to be allowed to die naturally should her heart stop beating. The decision was made just in time. A few days later, Posner discovers that Vivian has stopped breathing. In a panic, he mistakenly attempts to treat her, performing cardiopulmonary resuscitation (CPR) and calling for a crash cart. Susie tries to intervene but Posner won't listen. Eventually, Susie succeeds in explaining that Vivian had chosen to be DNR. Realising his mistake, Posner stops and steps back. Vivian dies. Even in her final moments, Vivian's life is intertwined with, and subject to, the nuances of communication and miscommunication.

On the theatre stage, after dying, Vivian walks away from her hospital bed, as if she were stepping into an afterlife. An individual restored, rather than a lesson taught.

3.10 *Mom's Cancer*[10]—Brian Fies

It is not forbidden to laugh with cancer patients—or even to laugh *at* them. In describing his mother's encounter with the disease, cartoonist Brian Fies provides us with many incidents worth laughing at. "Can you tell what caused it?" Fies's mother asks her doctor about her illness. "In my experience," the doctor replies, "one of five things." Counting on her fingers, she goes on to explain: "Smoking, smoking, smoking, smoking, or smoking."

Deep into her treatment, the woman phones the hospital. "I have a headache", she says, worried that this might mean something. The doctor

[10] For a recent edition, see: Fies, B. (2023). *Mom's Cancer*. New York: Abrams Comic Arts.

on the line fobs her off: "Yeah, don't worry about it." At her next visit to the hospital, she mentions also having had a cough, presuming that this too was trivial. "What?" the doctor exclaims. "You should have called at once!" Back home, now on high alert, the woman phones the hospital as soon as she feels tingling in her head. "That's normal with a brain tumour," comes the reply. In other words: *stop overreacting*. At her next appointment, she mentions a minor leg cramp. The doctor places hands-on-hips and berates her: "That could be a deadly blood clot! Why didn't you call?!" The next day, another phone call: "I can't breathe." The next response: "So? You have lung cancer! What'd you expect?" The cycle of misunderstanding is comedic: each ending is followed by another ending. Whenever she complains, she is told she is wrong. And when she doesn't complain, well, that's wrong too.

"How am I supposed to know?" she asks herself. After a while, she just stops contacting the hospital entirely.

The woman—Fies just calls her 'Mom'—lives at home, where she is cared for by her family. For most cancer patients, this is how they mainly live their lives. Hospital visits break the routine, immersing the patient in the midst of crowds of other people just like them, each with their own cancer story. The suddenness of social contact can provoke a rush of sharing. Even medical interns, in white coats for barely a few weeks, will describe being shocked at what patients entrust to them in conversation.

Mom is 66 years old, and has been diagnosed with lung cancer with metastases to the brain. She smoked all her adult life (hence her doctor's earlier enumeration) but is determined to 'conquer' her cancer. The narrator, her son, is in his early forties, and works as a cartoonist. To him, cartooning is a worldview as much as a genre. Every experience has the potential for humour.

Like most cancer patients, Mom is no oncologist! Her understanding of her illness is patchy to say the least. She is worried about whether or not to exercise while ill: "But what if I speed up my blood flow and it moves brain tumour cells to some other part of my body?" she wonders. "I don't think it works like that," replies her son. But in reality he's no oncologist either.

It is Mom's children who try to help their Mom to make sense of things. "At least it's just a Stage Four", Mom reassures herself, falsely believing that there are ten such stages. Not even up to halfway yet, she believes. "You know Stage Four is *bad*, right?" responds the son. Mom is taken aback and tries to reconfigure things: "So 'Stage Four' means they found cancer in four places…?" "No, Mom," say the children, frustrated because they have explained all this many times before (Levinsen et al., in press).

Whether right or wrong on the facts, Mom is determined to stay upbeat, delicately balancing denial with optimism (Czerwiec and Huang 2017). "You know, I think my scan tomorrow is a win-win," she muses, "if it shows the chemo's working and the cancer is shrinking, good for me. And if it shows the chemo's *not* working and the cancer's *not* responding, then I don't have to do any more chemo. I can't lose!"

Ultimately, her fortunes match her endurance. After all the appointments, the family meetings, the oxygen cylinders, the chemicals, the mingling with other cancer patients who smoke cigarettes before entering the radiation room, Mom's treatments end positively. The cancer is gone. The chemo *did* work. Mom didn't lose.

After all their travails, the family's celebrations are subdued. On the pages of the graphic novel, the illustrations turn from monochrome to full colour. Mom is shown moving house, as if physically leaving her cancer behind to go live apart from her illness. "Mom always wanted to live in Southern California," Fies explains. "I guess she figured it was now or never."

And yet even then, this ending is followed by another ending. At the very end of *Mom's Cancer*, Fies has added a short epilogue, which was hastily added just as the book was going to press. Six months after the original afterword was written, Mom passed away in her new home in California. Free of cancer, she died from medical complications that partly arose from her extensive post-cancer treatments. The steroids used to control inflammation in her brain had weakened her body, but reducing the dose ended up causing pressure in a different part of her brain, with fatal consequences. But she never regretted her choices. Aggressive treatment had given her two years of life that she would not otherwise have enjoyed, and, according to her children, she was never happier than when living in her new Hollywood home.

Mom's Cancer exploits cartooning to provide a fresh genre of literature and medicine: illness narratives in graphic form (Green and Myers 2010). In an appealing blend of text and images, Fies shows us how patients and their families navigate the disease trajectories that await them, and how understandings—*and misunderstandings*—of cancer form integral parts of the journey.

Such coping with cancer is a universal human endeavour: Fies's book has been translated into German, French, Italian, and Japanese. The iconography of illness is intuitively appealing to patients, and helps to transcend the gap between knowledge and fear. Getting patients to draw pictures of their cancer is not merely an aesthetic exercise, it is a pedagogical form of art therapy. The process helps patients to convey and to consolidate an understanding of the illness inside their bodies (Broadbent et al. 2019). Visual stories not only help orient patients to illness, they also frame matters for doctors and care professionals.

Conveniently, *Mom's Cancer* is a compact little volume. It fits neatly into a white coat pocket.

3.11 *A Journey Round My Skull*[11]—Frigyes Karinthy

It is not only doctors who produce diagnoses. Laypeople whose bodies (or minds) refuse to function as they would like to do so too. They end up ever on the lookout for signs of possible illness, poring over books about disease, searching online for stories about similar symptoms, and endlessly interrogating any fellow sufferers they happen to encounter. In this age of public health campaigns, self-examination, and mass screening, those who ignore the early warning signs of disease are liable to end up victim-blamed for their procrastination and dissimulation. And yet the more a concerned person researches their potential illnesses, the

[11] For a recent edition, see: Karinthy, F. (2008). *A Journey Round My Skull*. New York: New York Review of Books Classics.

greater their chances of being labelled a 'hypochondriac'. The problem is that subjective experiences of 'symptoms' do not always run parallel to objective reality. Such divergence of perception can produce fascinating reactions, even amongst medical care providers.

In his medical memoir *A Journey Round My Skull*, Hungarian writer Frigyes Karinthy (1887–1938) describes some truly bizarre symptoms, such as when he 'hears' a train departing even though he is nowhere near a railway. The noises exist only inside his head. Karinthy soon realises he is hallucinating. His ears in particular fool him, so much so that he cannot understand his friends in a Budapest restaurant. Somewhat aware of how organic brains can sometimes fail, Karinthy understands that he hasn't actually gone mad. Echoing Descartes, he logically concludes that "in that event, I should be incapable of diagnosing my case" (p. 14). Instead he visits an ENT doctor, who diagnoses a simple ear infection.

But the auditory hallucinations persist. Karinthy begins to find them amusing, pondering the punctuality of this invisible railway system and whether all the trains will ever reach their destinations. Unsatisfied with the ENT specialist, Karinthy visits a psychoanalyst. True to form, the Freudian attributes the auditory illusions to dysfunctions in Karinthy's early childhood experiences. But before the author can undergo formal analysis, new strange things start to happen. A mirror opposite him begins to move. Concluding that he might have a brain tumour, Karinthy visits his primary care physician. The sceptical doctor knows better, attributing his strange experiences to nicotine poisoning. Karinthy has only himself to blame for smoking too much.

Severe headaches and vomiting follow, and Karinthy becomes increasingly disoriented. Thinking that abnormalities in his vision might be a factor, he visits an ophthalmologist. But this person aggravates Karinthy with his haughtiness. "I felt it was his place to satisfy my legitimate curiosity," Karinthy records, "and not mine to bow to his 'professional' reticence" (p. 45). In due course, Karinthy starts to lean to the left and his handwriting becomes illegible. Probably more than just his vision is askew.

The "journey" around Karinthy's skull involves a battalion of doctors who end up searching for a diagnosis in or around the author's head (Frank 1991). As well as the ENT specialist, psychoanalyst, ophthalmologist, and primary care doctor, the expedition is eventually joined by oncologists, neurosurgeons, and neurologists (one of whom happens to be his own wife). Karinthy's increasingly strange symptoms produce an ever-changing array of signposts and landmarks, greatly complicating the logistics (Tsiakiri et al. 2025).

Karinthy's friends participate in the exploration. Some are optimistic and minimise his complaints, although Karinthy feels that they are doing so out of fear: "They are hiding their panic over the great mystery that awaits us all." Other friends are more serious. Some are simply businesslike, boldly asking Karinthy not to forget them in his will.

When the diagnosis is finally made—a tumour in the cerebellum—the doctors agree that Karinthy should be referred to Herbert Olivecrona in Stockholm, one of the best surgeons available (Olivecrona had studied in America under the legendary brain surgery pioneer, Harvey Cushing; Ljunggren 1993). Just before being admitted into surgery, Karinthy experiences a Biblical hallucination, featuring his skull and its tumour on the hill of Calvary. The operation itself is experienced surreally, the scalp incisions feeling like tiny pricks, the drilling of his skull numbing his ears, and various cracking sounds filling his mind, as though he were walking across creaking plank after creaking plank. During the operation, the surgeon politely inquires: "How are you feeling now?" "Thank you, professor, I'm fine," Karinthy replies, his head clamped in a steel structure and his brain exposed to the air.

The operation is a success. Suddenly, Karinthy can taste food again. His neurologist wife's fear that he would go blind turns out to be unjustified. The patient returns home, "like a shipwrecked man to whom a wave has offered the bounty of life's remaining years" (Bishop 1994).

The quest around his skull completed, Karinthy's life became gratifyingly banal once again.

3.12 *In Gratitude*[12]—Jenny Diski

The English author Jenny Diski (1947–2016) does not like playing hide and seek. Even in the first sentences of *In Gratitude*, her valedictory memoir, she defies cliché. When the doctor reveals her lung cancer diagnosis,

[12] For a recent edition, see: Diski, J. (2016). *In Gratitude*. London: Bloomsbury.

she feels "embarrassment, at first, to the exclusion of all other feelings" (p. 8). Embarrassment at the prospect of being given a role so familiar to her, a role so widely portrayed in popular culture that she knows what to expect despite never having had a relevant personal experience—the role of a cancer patient.

When she asks how long she might survive were she to undergo treatment—"I'm sure it's different for everyone, and only based on statistics, but could you perhaps give me a general idea: years…months …weeks?" (p. 13)—she feels panic set in, as her own meandering sentence structure slowly clarifies how short the time frame might actually be. She notes how the doctor is careful to phrase that part of his plan as "to treat, not to cure" (p. 14).

Diski was 66 years old at the time of diagnosis. Her life history colours her reaction. As a child, she had an absent and womanising father, and an alcoholic mother who touched her daughter's body inappropriately at bedtime ["What's the matter? There's nothing wrong. I'm your mother. You're still my little girl" (p. 25)]. Diski originally ran away from home and from school, and ended up in foster care. She was raped at the age of 14. Later, she was taken in by the mother of a school friend, who just happened to be the Nobel-winning novelist Doris Lessing. Lessing proved an intellectually inspiring mentor, standing in unrecognisable contrast with Diski's own parents.

Unsurprisingly, Diski was hardened by her life, but also became somewhat bitter and defensive. Her response to cancer is to assert herself, to go her own way about things and to "avoid the cancer clichés". She decries the idea of a 'bucket list' ("Really, there is nothing that I want to do before I die, except perhaps just lie back and enjoy the morphine…"; p. 18). She admonishes those around her: "Under no circumstances is anyone to say that I lost a battle with cancer. Or that I bore it bravely. I am not fighting, losing, winning or bearing" (p. 18). She rejects the rhetorical habit of personifying cancer cells as animate adversaries that can be challenged or resisted by patients (Kaptein and Thong 2018; Sisi et al. 2025; Timmermann 2014). "I reject all metaphors of attack or enmity in the midst", she writes. Diski cannot help but notice that her commitment to rejecting the clichés of cancer itself perversely requires her *to focus on them even more*. Like it or not, she is locked into this journey, clichés, and all.

The middle part of the book is entitled 'Chemo and Me', and is sandwiched between her chaotic childhood and her recollections of adult life as an author, critic, journalist, and partner. Cancer should not take centre stage, she feels. Nonetheless, she experiences amnesia, a cascade of typos when writing, and a fear of falling down stairs. Not to mention fatigue: "Fatigue isn't more tired than tiredness," she notes, "it's differently tired…your veins imploded and sucked dry by a monstrous gravity" (p. 97). Getting into a car is only possible with a sip of morphine and a handheld fan (Hamann et al. 2018a).

In the chemotherapy rooms, she focuses on the clinical care staff, whom she refers to as *Onc Doc* and *Onc Nurse*. She tries to ignore the other patients "because people in various stages of cancer treatment aren't a group anyone wants to be a part of" (p. 100). At radiotherapy, the technicians press her body into the "death ray" equipment, precisely to the millimetre. Although her breasts are bare, the lab technician carelessly removes the gown that covers her nudity while walking from the changing room to the treatment table. Diski describes her treatment with the "death rays": the steel arms of the machinery humming, clicking, and twisting, sweeping unexpectedly as if suddenly going the wrong way. She becomes afraid that the machine will collapse and crush her (Kaptein et al. 2025).

Within range of diagnostic predictions, Diski died at the age of 69. She had received her own copy of *In Gratitude* just six days earlier, on her sickbed.

Like many writers, Diski became intrigued by the discourse of cancer. At one point she is told that she has "non-small cell lung adenocarcinoma" (p. 119). But why did the doctors use this strange term, *non-small*? "Why not 'large' or 'quite big'?" she asks, quite reasonably. It reminds her of how in *The Pit and the Pendulum*, Edgar Allen Poe's narrator spoke about a character having "unclosed my eyes". She concludes that such linguistic devices might serve a survival function. They might help distract us from the horrible.

3.13 *Intoxicated By My Illness*[13]—Anatole Broyard

Anatole Broyard (1920–1990) was an author and a renowned literary critic, who wrote daily book reviews for the *New York Times* for 15 years. He also was an editor at the *New York Review of Books*. Such was his stature, he was widely seen as a gatekeeper of New York literature. Although acknowledged as a superlative writer in his own right, and despite having produced hundreds of columns and articles, his own two books were not published until after he had died. One of these, *Intoxicated By My Illness*, relays the story of the final episode of his life.

Broyard spent his life traversing thresholds of reality. Born into a Black family in Louisiana, he moved with his parents to New York at the height of the Great Depression. He and his sister had a distinctly lighter skin tone than the rest of the family. As a result, Anatole was bullied not only by the local white kids, who were aware of his Black heritage, but also by the Black children he encountered—because he "looked white" (B. Broyard 2007). Later in life, Broyard would become increasingly ambiguous about his own ethnic identity (Gates, Jr. 1996). When he joined the army, he completed officer training, despite the fact such training was effectively restricted to white enlistees. As recorded in his daughter's memoir, he kept his ethnic ancestry a secret from his own children (B. Broyard 2007). And in developing his writing career, he avoided identifying with or championing themes of Black identity. As the author Brent Staples would later observe, Broyard just wanted to be a writer; he didn't want to end up "consigned to the back of the literary bus" (Staples 2003).

Broyard's ability to subvert expectations carried through into his account of prostate cancer. In explaining the illness that would eventually kill him, Broyard denies being hampered or debilitated. On the contrary, he describes being inspired and intoxicated by his disease. "So much of a writer's life consists of assumed suffering," he records. "I felt something like relief, even elation, when the doctor told me that I had cancer…"

[13] For a recent edition, see: Broyard, A. (1993). *Intoxicated By My Illness: And Other Writings on Life and Death*. New York: Random House.

(p. 3). Broyard notes that people often try to flee from such a diagnosis. He, on the other hand, "turned toward it" (p. 3).

A key message can be found in Broyard's chapter on medical consultations, which, in a characteristic contraposition, is entitled *The Patient Examines the Doctor*. This is no treatise on the invasiveness of diagnostics, chemotherapy, or radiation, or on the indignities of rectal examinations and erectile dysfunction. Broyard does not focus on pain or sadness. Instead, he turns everything around. He produces a set of commandments for good medical care. Broyard seeks to set out how things should be ideally done in medicine (Xiang et al. 2025).

In Broyard's view, a good doctor needs to be capable of more than physical examinations. An effective medical investigator, he feels, "has to get to my character." Such a doctor "has to go through my soul," he writes. "He doesn't only have to go through my anus" (p. 40). Broyard also recommends that doctors try to see through a patient's surface cheerfulness in order to detect their inner panic. What can seem routine to a doctor on their rounds can be a life-changing crisis for a person with cancer.

Not that Broyard feels doctors should devote unending time to interacting with patients. Instead, quality matters more than quantity. Broyard recommends that doctors need not do more than focus on a patient's situation "for perhaps five minutes"; what is important is that they do it *seriously*. Doctors should give their "whole mind" to a patient at least once. After all, "each man is ill in his own way" (p. 44). In this manner, Broyard emphasises the importance of authentic availability.

Overall, Broyard emphasises the need for doctors and patients to see each other as equals, a view perhaps reflecting the author's own encounters with arbitrary prejudicial hierarchy. He wants doctors to "enjoy" being with their patients, to be *interesting to* the patient as well as *interested in* them, and to acknowledge that, as regular human beings with their own strengths and aptitudes, patients will in some respects be *superior* to their doctors, rather than naturally subordinate to them.

Mostly, Broyard wants doctors and patients to empathise with each other. "Physicians have been taught in medical school that they must keep the patient at a distance", he writes. "A doctor's job would be so much more interesting and satisfying if he simply let himself plunge into the patient…" (p. 49).

Radiotherapy and chemotherapy kept Broyard going for around a year, providing him with a reasonable quality of life. Nonetheless, he lived just for a few weeks after being hospitalised. The manuscript for *Intoxicated By My Illness* was finalised by Broyard's wife, Sandy, who looked after its eventual publication.

In many respects, Broyard's views on medical care were decades ahead of their time. The idea that doctors should seek to establish personal connections with patients—rather than to assiduously avoid them—has recently re-emerged as a priority for enlightened medical practice. As such, Broyard's book would make excellent training material for medical education (Florijn et al. 2019). In 2020, the American Medical Association published a special review in *JAMA* detailing five evidence-based methods that doctors can use to establish "physician presence" and "connection with patients" during clinical encounters, all with the aim of maximising the efficacy of clinical care (Zulman et al. 2020). These five methods—*prepare for meaningful interaction*, *listen intently and completely*, *agree on what matters*, *connect with the patient's story*, and *explore emotional cues*—strongly echo the advice offered by Broyard some 30 years previously.

Human psychology is primed towards tribalism and hierarchy. In a world of in-groups and out-groups, marginalisation and supremacy, and the embedding of structural power, sometimes what is needed most is someone, like Anatole Broyard, to remind us that *all* perspectives are worthy of challenge, *all* the time.

Cancer patients should not be defined by their illness at the expense of their humanity. And, as participants in the healthcare system, they should not assume to belong at the back of the bus.

3.14 *A Very Easy Death*[14]—Simone de Beauvoir

Simone de Beauvoir (1908–1986) famously did not see her work as amounting to 'philosophy', but she nonetheless became acclaimed as one of the leading existentialist philosophers of her generation. Philosophers consider *A Very Easy Death*, her autobiographical novella, to be one of the more extreme literary depictions of existentialism ever written. Partially inspired by her life companion Jean-Paul Sartre, with whom she had an open relationship for more than 50 years, Beauvoir uses *A Very Easy Death* to emphasise to readers that an individual themselves is the only one who can give meaning to their own existence. This is as true, if not truer, when that individual is gravely ill.

In *A Very Easy Death*, de Beauvoir offers a detailed account of the final life stages of her mother, who died from cancer in 1963. A recurring theme relates to the dilemmas of disclosure in serious disease, the ethics of truth-telling when interacting with the terminally ill. De Beauvoir also describes her discomfort at being surprised at her own emotional reactions to her mother's demise. Before, de Beauvoir had felt she had little emotional connection to her mother, but once the woman became ill, her impulses changed.

Notably, de Beauvoir had previously achieved fame for her critique of motherhood itself, having called for a revolution in how society sees women's humanity. In *The Second Sex*, which appeared in 1949, de Beauvoir argued that the biology of motherhood was banal rather than profound, that the mysticising of childbirth was thus an arbitrary restriction on women's autonomy, and that culture should therefore supersede nature in order for women to be truly existentially free.

In *A Very Easy Death*, de Beauvoir describes how doctors and nurses bear heavy burdens of medical responsibility (Elsner 2019). Even when the mother is juggling life with death, those around her resist discussing the full details of her diagnosis or prognosis. De Beauvoir reflects on the 'ease' of her mother's "upper-class death", being well looked after in

[14] For a recent edition, see: de Beauvoir, S. (1985). *A Very Easy Death*. New York: Pantheon.

hospital. The daughter's discomfort at having neglected their relationship becomes more acute as the older woman declines. "When someone you love dies," de Beauvoir concludes, "you pay for the sin of outliving her with a thousand piercing regrets" (p. 94).

The events of *A Very Easy Death* will be familiar to oncologists. De Beauvoir's mother, a 77-year-old woman, falls in the bathroom and breaks her leg. When repairing the hip, an orthopaedic surgeon suspects that more than just the bone is broken, and after further medical examinations, the woman is diagnosed with colorectal cancer. The internists and oncologists do not consider further active treatment worthwhile, and the patient dies after just a few weeks.

Initially, de Beauvoir represents the doctors harshly: "Dr J, Professor B, Dr T: neat, trim, shining, well-groomed, bending over this ill-kempt, rather wild-looking old woman from an immense height" (p. 21). The daughter resists the doctors' paternalism, aghast that Professor B would promise that her mother will soon be able to "potter around" again. De Beauvoir is horrified that this was how the doctors viewed women in their seventies: old ladies good for little more than "pottering" (Back 2020).

The medical procedures continue, gastric tubes are inserted, and surgery reveals metastatic colon cancer. The patient is told she has peritonitis. De Beauvoir questions why the doctor would persist in "tormenting" her mother when it is clear she is going to die. The doctor replies that he is "doing what has to be done." But even the nurses are sceptical, telling de Beauvoir to refuse any further operations (Ding et al. 2025).

De Beauvoir contrasts the paternalism she saw in medicine with the history of her own upbringing under the influence of her mother, seeing beyond the woman's state as "a living corpse". She concludes that while it is often observed that parents do not understand their children very well, the opposite is also true: children are fundamentally disconnected from their parents. The banality of childbirth as described in *The Second Sex*—the fact that women do not really "make" children, but merely allow their flesh to engender more flesh—serves to emphasise the separateness of parent and child, a feminist argument modified by its existential implications. Forever separate, human beings are inherently existentially lonely. In its own way, this state of things makes the doctors' arrogance more striking, and de Beauvoir begins to appreciate their paternalism as insofar as it is preferable to ambivalence. Eventually, the mother dies at night, while de Beauvoir is resting at home. Although de Beauvoir herself is shaken by the event, the doctors, nurses, and daughter herself are comforted by the fact that the mother has died a somewhat "easy" death.

The paternalism observed by de Beauvoir in the 1960s is often cited as a feature of medical history, rather than part of its present. However, women continue to report very different experiences of healthcare compared to men, and many statistical datasets reveal worrying trends of sex differences in medical outcomes. In that regard, the themes of *A Very Easy Death* continue to resonate today.

Existentialism flourished in the nineteenth and twentieth centuries, and often no longer seems fashionable among philosophers, never mind medical students. However, meaning and responsibility in illness and suffering continue to be priorities for patients and their families. Our dread and anxiety in the face of death—and their bringing into view of the meaninglessness of existence itself—remain important to consider as we evaluate the merits of medical interventions and treatments.

3.15 *Mortality*[15]—Christopher Hitchens

The philosopher John Gray once described the Anglo-American essayist Christopher Hitchens (1949–2011) as "one of the greatest living writers of English prose" (Gray 2011); after Hitchens had passed away, journalist Alexander Linklater commented that "the only word of that which is certainly untrue is that Hitchens is no longer living" (Linklater 2012). Hitchens died in 2011 from complications associated with oesophageal cancer. His posthumously published book, *Mortality*, features a series of essays the author had published when describing his struggles with illness during the final year of his life.

Hitchens is often characterised as a contrarian, a writer who takes the opposing view almost as a matter of course. Famously atheistic, he frequently wrote about the limits of philosophising about one's own

[15] For a recent edition, see: Hitchins, C. (2012). *Mortality*. New York: Twelve.

afterlife. For him, death is final and something to be approached *rationally* (Brennan 2018).

Hitchens's time was divided between the United Kingdom, where he spent the first half of his life, and the United States, where he lived from his thirties onward. Forthrightly polemical, he wrote prodigiously on politics, economics, war, religion, and culture. His works were widely acclaimed and, at times, widely condemned.

Mortality begins with Hitchens waking up in a New York hotel the morning after a boozy book launch: "The whole cave of my chest and thorax seemed to have been hollowed out and then refilled with slow-drying cement" (p. 1). As he observes, this is not the first time he had woken up "feeling like death" (p. 1). But on this occasion, the metaphor nudges towards reality. After he is taken to a clinic by an emergency medical team called by the hotel, the doctors find shadows in his X-rays. They tell him he should see an oncologist. At first, Hitchens goes into denial. He continues about his day, appears on a television show as planned, and later participates in a sold-out literary event with Salman Rushdie. No one notices anything amiss, even though Hitchens is violently ill before both engagements.

But his denial stage is short-lived. He likens his transition from *healthy* to *cancer-stricken* to a migrant travelling to "the sick country" while emotionally "clinging to their old domicile" (p. 3). Echoing political narratives around the realities of migration, Hitchens describes the "new land" in which he finds himself. "The country has a language of its own – a lingua franca that manages to be both dull and difficult…as well as some unsettling gestures that require a bit of getting used to." For example: "an official met for the first time may abruptly sink his fingers into your neck." Indeed, it was one such physical examination that revealed Hitchens's cancer to have spread to his lymph nodes. He names this new land *Tumorville*. Its motto: "Tissue is the issue" (p. 3).

Hitchens considers contrarianism to be a constructive part of dialogue. In his view, division should not be demonised. After all, what would be the point of politics if everyone agreed on everything? Contrarianism forces people to evaluate their assumptions, and so is essential to findings resolutions. Unsurprisingly, therefore, when Hitchens applies his contrarianist approach to cancer, one of the first things he challenges is its clichés.

True to form, Hitchens focuses on the more profound examples. The classic inquiry of cancer patients—"Why me?"—he dismisses as an especially "dumb" question. In his view, the natural reply (from "the cosmos") should be simple: "Why not?" (p. 3).

He turns the stereotype of patients "battling against" cancer on its head. "I'm not fighting or battling cancer," he argues. "It's fighting me" (p. 87). All the time, his cancer is on manoeuvres, its only mission to destroy his body, and, with it, his life. Even while he sleeps, he is under attack (Florijn et al. 2019; Hauser and Schwarz 2020; Sowell et al. 2025).

If Hitchens is resolved to engage with any enemy, it is with obscurantism: cancer-related alternative medicine, pseudoscience, and religious fundamentalism. Hitchens is especially galled at the prospect of being "prayed for." To support his point he cites a 2006 research study published in the *American Heart Journal.* Having conducted a randomised controlled trial on more than 1200 patients, the researchers had found no association between being "prayed for" and surgery outcomes. Patients who were prayed for fared no better than patients who were not (Benson et al. 2006). In fact, patients who *knew* that someone was praying for them tended to do slightly *worse*, possibly because they were more likely to lose motivation when complications arose. It was as though they would feel *guilty* at having disappointed the people who prayed for them.

Hitchens explains how positive thinking often carries such a downside. He tells how his friends reassure him that "If anyone can beat this, you can", the phrase itself standing as another cancer cliché. Other supporters convey similar messages. They are convinced that death itself will be no match for the great Christopher Hitchens: "Cancer has no chance against someone like you" (p. 18). The problem, though, is that such reassurances do not allow for defeat. Meeting battle-cry metaphors with attributions of heroism sets cancer patients up for failure. "On bad days, and even on better ones, such exhortations can have a vaguely depressing effect," Hitchens observes. "If I check out, I'll be letting all these comrades down" (p. 18). He much prefers a more sombre approach. He proposes an etiquette in which there is no veiled language or obscuring of misery: "I'll do the facing of hard facts, thanks. Don't you be doing it too"

(p. 39). When asked by friends how he is doing, he develops a habit of replying cryptically: "A bit early to say" (p. 40).

Mortality reaches its poignant climax with two unorthodox final chapters. The first is a series of fragmentary thoughts collated from unfinished writings that Hitchens left behind when he died. Hitchens notes the irony of his specific form of cancer: a polemicist whose voice had often been condemned as blasphemous, now struck down by cancer of the oesophagus. He wonders if he will live to see the expiration date on his credit card. The final chapter is an afterword written by his wife, the screenwriter Carol Blue. "Onstage," she writes, "my husband was an impossible act to follow" (p. 95). And yet now she must follow him. But Christopher still manages to have the last word: Carol describes how she keeps discovering notes and jottings that Hitchens has left behind in their home, in stacks of papers "on surfaces all around the apartment", in unpacked suitcases brought back from travelling, and inside the back covers of books, neatly inserted to preserve a thought for some future writing project. "At any time," she writes, she can therein "peruse our library or his notes and rediscover and recover him" (p. 102).

In an extended television interview recorded shortly before his death (see https://youtu.be/LIVEsa2g4ag), Hitchens emphasised the distinction between "death" and "dying." The latter can, and should, be feared, he argued. But the former—the state of "being dead"—should frighten no one, because no one can have feelings about *anything* when they are dead. Including about their own existence.

In accordance with his wishes, after he died Hitchens's body was donated to medical research. For Hitchens, an afterlife is something to which the deceased are eternally oblivious—but which nonetheless retains a moral dimension.

3.16 *The Cancer Journals*[16]—Audre Lorde

In *The Cancer Journals,* Audre Lorde describes her exasperation with modern cancer care. Urged by a nurse to wear a prosthetic bra following her mastectomy, she is wholly uncomfortable at the idea. Her retelling of

[16] For a recent edition, see: Lorde, A. (2020). *The Cancer Journals*. London: Penguin.

the nurse's words reveals a multiplicity of medical motivations for the recommendation, not all of which could be described as patient-centred. "We really like you to wear something, at least when you come in [to the clinic]", the nurse points out. "Otherwise it's bad for the morale of the office" (p. 59).

Audre Lorde is often described as many things: she was a writer, a civil rights activist, a philosopher, and a professor, among many other formal roles. But beyond these occupations, she was other things too. She famously described herself as a "Black, lesbian, feminist, socialist, mother, warrior, poet" (Lorde 1983). She also adhered to "womanism", a broader, more socialist form of feminism that sought to bypass racial stereotypes in the feminist movement and take account of Black women's experiences (Olson 2011).

We might say that this was very much Lorde's own position: she never held herself within one single identity, but as the epitome of an intersectional person. Once she had cancer, she acquired further identities extending into illness and disability, those of the patient. In several respects, her medical encounters were problematic for precisely the reason that clinicians struggled to see her for who she fully was. They failed to recognise the many sides to her being. [As authors, we are especially keen to acknowledge our own positionality within this discussion. It is difficult, if not impossible, for us as two white European men to properly encapsulate Lorde's experiences or perspectives, and our observations here will inevitably be constrained by this cultural distance. We intend here to write with deference to Lorde's own words and statements.]

The nurse's insistence on prosthetic bras is an epiphany in Lorde's journey, and her cancer was in many ways a stimulus for her activist thinking. She embraces the fight metaphor, so fiercely rejected by others (such as Susan Sontag; as discussed in the chapter on Sontag in this book). "I refuse to have my scars hidden or trivialized behind lambswool or silicone gel," she declares. "…I refuse to hide my body simply because it might make a woman-phobic world more comfortable" (p. 60).

Lorde's medical history had been rather unremarkable for a woman in whom breast cancer was diagnosed, although she would perhaps hate this biomedical framing. Her first biopsy sample had indicated a benign growth in her breast, but a few weeks later the diagnosis is revised:

malignant tissue in her right breast. Her warrior ethos leads her to actively seek support from other women, with and without cancer. She gives a voice to her cancer, by talking and writing about the fear of its recurrence, her quest to integrate illness and its medical management into her daily life. Breast cancer, she writes in her diary, "can still be a gateway", allowing for "the tapping and expansion of my own power and knowing" (p. 54).

Lorde entertains emotions that some health psychologists would label as denial or wishful thinking ("I'm so tired of all this. I want to be the person I used to be, the real me. I feel sometimes that it's all a dream and surely I'm about to wake up now"; p. 25). Ultimately, her story does not end well, and she dies a decade later as a consequence of her illness. In her desire for self-control she turns to complementary treatment modalities, all the time seeking intensive support from other women. In this regard, her approach both resembles and differs from that of other feminist writers. Barbara Ehrenreich, for example, famously rebuked pseudoscientific and esoteric takes on cancer and its treatment, while sharing Lorde's deep scepticism of the mainstream cancer recovery 'industry', with all its ethos of positive thinking and other designations of 'correct' female responding (cf., Ehrenreich 2009).

Lorde committed her thoughts to personal diaries, which poignantly present the personal in a private voice (albeit one so smoothly written as to allow for eventual publication). In this regard, she intuitively sought the benefits of so-called expressive writing interventions, the benefits of which have since been explored in an extensive body of empirical work (see Kaptein 2022; Körner et al. 2019; Watson et al. 2025; Wu et al. 2025). For Lorde, this act of recording further augmented her identity. She describes the experience of cancer as not merely biomedical or physical, but as one that requires "physical and psychic nourishment to repair past and minimise future damage to [her] body" (p. 16). But even so, in Lorde's estimation, not everything psychological is automatically supreme. Some bodily experiences, such as pain, can be overwhelming. "I had thought the emotional and psychological pain would be the worst," she recalls, "but it was the physical pain that seemed to be doing me in" (p. 38). The capacity of the body to displace the spirit was unavoidable.

"The physical pain was power," she continued, "for it kept that conscious part of me away from the full flavour of my fear and loss" (p. 39).

Such consideration of how physical experience intrudes into subjective mental life extends far beyond the rudimentary elemental depictions offered even by the biopsychosocial model. Perhaps, therefore, we could add yet another role to Lorde's interlocking identities: that of astute psychological theorist (Diouri et al. 2025).

3.17 *Clock Without Hands*[17]—Carson McCullers

A clock without hands, when tattooed on a prisoner's wrist, is intended to represent a long sentence. For people with cancer, a clock without hands can represent life itself, in which time emotionally stands still. Carson McCullers's (1917–1967) own life was relatively short-lived. In old photographs, the American writer looks shy and small, but she was known to be an assertive speaker. Her books, too, spoke loudly, if often indirectly. McCullers explored spiritual themes of belonging and loneliness, in-groups and eccentricity, and the nature of isolation within crowds. Writing in the Deep South of the United States in the 1940s and 1950s, she would often depict her characters as being heart-broken by the unachievability of love (the film adaptation of her novel *Reflections in a Golden Eye* cast Marlon Brando and Elizabeth Taylor as embroiled in an especially fraught sexual relationship). Many scholars point to her persistent hinting at gay and lesbian themes, suggesting that she "camouflaged her love for women" in her writing (Whitt 1999, p. 134).

As a young girl, McCullers devoured anything that was legible. As a woman, she ran into relationship problems with an alcoholic and apparently latently homosexual husband—who was eventually to take his own life and invite her to do the same. McCullers developed an addiction to alcohol, had multiple strokes, and eventually developed breast cancer (Oates 2017). In her novels, these arduous experiences translated into a deep insight into people's feelings and behaviours.

[17] For a recent edition, see: McCullers, C. (2008). *Clock Without Hands*. London: Penguin.

In a poem dedicated to McCullers, the poet Charles Bukowski recalled "all her books of terrified loneliness" (2007). Singer-songwriter Suzanne Vega based her entire 2016 album *Lover, Beloved* on Carson's life story, having been inspired by McCullers since she first read her novels at the age of 15. In the song *Carson's Blues,* Vega has McCullers cry out: "You've got to understand, understand, understand/That I've never belonged."

McCullers's life history colours her portrayal of cancer in *Clock Without Hands*. Her keen eye captures life in Milan, Georgia, and the United States more broadly, in and around 1950. The atmosphere of the novel is warm, stuffy, and rural. There is much racial discrimination, as well as hatred of those Northerners who dare come to "the South" to start a new life (Brennan 2012). A judge and a pharmacist, local dignitaries, are two of the main characters. On Sunday mornings, they gather after church with other important men to drink whiskey and smoke cigars. The 40-year-old pharmacist, Malone (an echo of "I'm alone") develops fatigue, loses his appetite, and finds that his suits are becoming loose around his body. Pulsating veins in his temples soon become visible. His doctor draws some blood, just to be sure. At the next appointment, once he is alone with the doctor, Malone immediately senses that something is amiss. The physician dares not look at him; his "familiar face seemed somehow eyeless."

The doctor continues to procrastinate by playing with a letter opener and eventually Malone has to break the silence, asking him what the tests have shown. "We have checked carefully and there seems to be something unusual in the blood chemistry," the doctor reports. The nervous Malone begins to chatter about anaemia, but the doctor cuts him off. "The white blood cells are abnormally increased…" he explains. "You probably understand what that means." But Malone does not understand at all. He could only *sense* what it means.

After a few more exchanges, and with Malone prevented from speaking by a thermometer placed in his mouth, the doctor gets to the point: "The long and short of it is, we have here a case of leukemia." After the examination, the doctor washes his hands. Malone finds that he is offended by this implication of his toxicity. He asks: "Well, how long do you give me, Doctor?" Only then does the doctor look him in the eye.

"I think we might count on a year or fifteen months," he suggests. Malone continues to babble nervously, and eventually breaks down in tears. The doctor responds to this emotionality with an appeal to empiricism—"Every month science discovers a new weapon against disease"—but Malone, a pharmacist, knows better than that. For him in this moment, it is the emotions that matter more (von Engelhardt 2021a; Riskin 2016).

Later Malone seeks comfort from his friend the judge, over a large glass of whiskey. "Leucocytes?" the judge queries. "Never heard of them." Malone explains that they are rather important but the judge is unconvinced. "If it was your heart or liver or even your kidneys," he advises, "I could understand your alarm." For the judge, the very fact that he has never heard of leucocytes makes them "seem a little far-fetched." They might not even exist. "I bet there's nothing wrong with you that sensible living and a spell of Milan summer won't cure," he opines, relying on a form of common-sense reasoning that psychologists often refer to as the availability heuristic: the tendency to believe that the familiar is far more powerful than the obscure (Moreno-Alonso et al. 2025).

The pharmacist drowns in his loneliness. He had asked his doctor for the truth, but really just wanted reassurance. And then the doctor went to wash his hands…

Eventually Malone's life ebbs away as he sits on a chair waiting for his wife to fetch a glass of water for him. To his wife, Malone's last breath sounds like a sigh. She stands there with the glass of water in her hand, the banality of death and the disconnections among the living highlighted once again. "Death is always the same," McCullers had written in the opening sentence of the novel, "but each man dies in his own way."

McCullers was a diminutive woman, but far from fragile. "A fallen deer, that's what they call me," Suzanne Vega had her sing, "But I'm an iron butterfly." Truly, her pen struck sharply as she explored the resilient isolation of human suffering and the primacy of heart over intellect. Patient Malone and writer McCullers were as one in their wisdom, and in their loneliness.

3.18 *When David Lost His Voice*[18]—Judith Vanistendael

In her graphic novel *When David Lost His Voice*, writer and artist Judith Vanistendael (1974–) writes as though she is breaking bad news. On page 2, the diagnosis is stated: supraglottic cancer of the larynx, Type T_3 N_{26} M_0. The doctor draws a head and a neck, with an intimidating black spot on the larynx. He places a red circle around it, and then an arrow pointing to the location of the tumour. David, the patient, disappears into a grey mist. Over a few pages, the narrative becomes surreal. Frame after frame, an angelic woman appears, bringing David a ball of golden light: "It's good against all sorts of troubles," she explains, "like pessimism, dark thoughts and depression." She places the golden orb into his chest. "Now, now, love," she says, "don't worry." David calls out to the woman in his hallucination. He addresses her as his "Nanny".

Vanistendael's story of the patient's life is dominated by women. David's daughter Miriam looks at her father and, to her horror, sees his face change into a mere skull with fuzzy grey outlines. Tamar, a grandchild, agrees with her boyfriend that she will mummify David, so that he can always stay with her. Paula, David's second wife, feels she is "a prisoner in a pitch-black room", imagining herself surrounded by dozens of scans of metastases on the walls of her apartment.

Vanistendael's book was inspired by the death of the author's own father-in-law. Across nearly 300 pages, she tells the story of how the ripples of cancer are felt through a patient's family network (Mäkitie et al. 2024). She skilfully exploits the capacity of graphics to tell a story using multiple modalities. The tenderness of her artwork is accentuated by her choice of watercolour. After David's larynx is surgically removed, the novel becomes predominantly nonverbal: we mostly have images, rendered in one or two colours, and largely devoid of speech bubbles. In this way, illustrations must also be 'read'. Colours and framing provide insight into the experience of being ill, by poignantly immersing the reader into the environment of the patient (Gibson et al. 2022).

[18] For a recent edition, see: Vanistendael, J. (2012). *When David Lost His Voice*. London: SelfMadeHero.

The form of a graphic novel provides the reader—a viewer—with an insight into how drawings can enrich medicine. Doctors can draw pictures to show patients what a disease is. Vanistendael even has David's own doctor do precisely this in the opening scene of *When David Lost His Voice*. Medical diagrams can often be quite mechanical, focusing less on the experience of being ill and more on the bits and pieces of the body that have gone awry. Advocates of 'graphic medicine' often discuss objectification as a gold standard for medical education and clinical care, something that complements biomedical thinking and action (Czerwiec et al. 2015). By contrast, patient drawings are often stylised in ways that convey a person's *feelings* about being sick (Broadbent et al. 2019; Jansen et al. 2019). Just as bibliotherapy (reading about being ill) and expressive writing (writing about being ill) allow a discourse to emerge in words, graphical drawing allows communication to expand far beyond the range of 'ordinary' medical expression (Kaptein et al. 2018).

After he loses his voice, David presents Miriam with a note saying "My darling, I am with you." She takes it home and places it in a small vial that she attaches to a necklace and hangs around her neck. Vanistendael shows the vial glowing warmly on Miriam's chest, exactly where David's Nanna had previously placed a golden orb of light. The glowing colour conveys something that words alone can't express.

Good against all sorts of troubles…like pessimism, dark thoughts, and depression.

3.19 *Stage Four*[19]—Sander Kollaard

While not unheard of, it is rare for ill people to refuse medical treatment. Alienation and irritation are not the usual responses. But sometimes a person can just end up overwhelmed. In *Stage Four*, a 2015 novel by Dutch author Sander Kollaard (1961–), the main character, Sarie, becomes frustrated in this manner. She complains that she wants to be left alone. "I don't want any more treatments," she cries, "and I don't want euthanasia" (p. 39).

[19] For a recent edition, see: Kollaard, S. (2018). *Stage Four: A Novel*. Seattle: AmazonCrossing.

Sarie had become ill while on a road trip with her husband, Barend. They had planned to revisit some of the places where they first fell in love in the 1960s, but now their vacation takes on a grim new dimension. When she was young, Sarie was inspired by ideals of equality and justice.

She and her husband had embarked on a journey into their past, to the Swedish island of Öland, but now face an uncertain future. Thoughts about lung cancer, and even the prospect of euthanasia, replace those of optimism, sun, and romance. The visit to Sweden foreshadowed these austere reflections. Allusions to the films of Ingmar Bergman feature frequently in the novel. Individuality and autonomy are recurring themes in Bergman's films, and also in Sarie's existence.

But now, diagnosed with Stage 4 non-small cell lung carcinoma at the age of 62, romance is exchanged for medication, carefully divided into five containers by her husband every day. The pills form an assortment of "reassuring pastel colours" (p. 80) and Barend at first takes pleasure in this task, whistling while he works. Guiltily realising his own moment of levity, Barend silences himself in case Sarie would hear him. But Sarie doesn't mind. "You were enjoying yourself. What's wrong with that?" she reassures her husband. "I enjoy sitting here, despite everything" (p. 81).

Stage Four is an unusual novel, in that it contains much carefully researched background information that the author presents in a didactic form. "Cancer is caused by uncontrolled cell division," begins one section, as if Kollaard is now writing a medical textbook. This is followed by paragraphs detailing the process of cell division, its regulation by DNA, and the way the symptoms of cancer manifest often indirectly. Kollaard describes the nature of exponential cell growth using numbers: showing how quickly the series *two, four, eight, sixteen…* progresses to *1024* (two to the power of ten), *32,768* (two to the power of fifteen), *1,048,576* (two to the power of twenty) and beyond.

At times, dramatic cancer imagery displaces scientific objectivity. Kollard frequently employs the standard medical metaphor where disease processes are imbued with a spirit of their own autonomy, a type of animism that attributes cells of the body with consciousness and intention: "Malignant cells break off all communication with their surroundings and spitefully force their way, slithering and sliding, through all possible tissues," he writes, "…blind and interested only in their own fruitless growth" (p. 23). Scientists often do this; they frequently describe inert objects as exhibiting purposeful action, belying the idea that they are truly inanimate (Hughes 2023). The shorthand of describing non-conscious things as pursuing particular objectives (such as "their own fruitless growth") is intended to be figurative rather than literal. However, in medical science, these metaphors are used so regularly that an important fact can often be forgotten: namely, that the underlying processes that are being described in this way *are not yet fully understood* (Riskin 2016).

The problem with animist metaphors is that they can lead to a form of determinism, a feeling that quasi-random events are in fact 'caused' by agents with deliberate intentions. Sarie sees her lung cancer as almost unavoidable, like a "meteorite on its way to destruction" (p. 105). But her husband sees it differently: "To Barend, cancer was not fate but an enemy, not an invading army but a treacherous platoon in one's own body. The diagnosis was not bad news but a declaration of war…" (p. 26). What Sarie saw as surrender, Barend saw as a challenge. Once again, the notion of autonomy looms large in this novel, even at the cellular level.

Kollaard lives and works in Sweden, a society often acknowledged for its culture of individuality. And yet this is a novel about relationships. Sarie and Barend's interactions draw attention to the huge toll that cancer can place on intimate couples (Fitch 2020; Kedia et al. 2019; Kaptein and Thong 2018; Kim E et al. 2025). Their dialogue is often perfunctory, but the characters' actions reveal underlying reams of human sentiment.

Sarie also feels deep solidarity with the many other patients she sees at the outpatient clinic, "driven out of the land of healthy people: a sickly tribe, wandering around the desert, without any reliable knowledge of their destination" (p. 35). She and her husband, she slowly realises, now belong to different tribes, placing the couple on opposite sides of a hidden border. "Perhaps this was why Barend annoyed her so much," Sarie reflects. Wife and husband are now speakers of different dialects.

Sarie ultimately epitomises the triumph of autonomy. She chooses to steer her own destiny. In her mind, even euthanasia involves succumbing to a process beyond her control, so she wishes to let nature, and cancer, take its course. Her penchant for self-determination pushes Barend to agree to her wish. She finds her death back on Öland. The author,

Kollaard, thereby himself sets out a path to death, one that occupies a unique place in the research literature on cancer and dying (Hamann et al. 2018a; Updike. 1982).

3.20 *The Crab in the Backseat*[20]—Élisabeth Gille

Élisabeth Gille (1937–1996) wrote three books, two of which were centred upon the horrors experienced by Jewish people during the Holocaust. Born Élisabeth Epstein in Paris in 1937, Gille survived the Second World War in hiding along with her sister. The girls' father, a banker, and their mother, the bestselling novelist Irène Némirovsky, were both deported to Auschwitz from France in 1942, where they died. Élisabeth's first book was an account of her mother's life, written in a semi-fictionalised autobiographical voice. Her third book was a novel about a Jewish girl who spent the war with her sister in a Catholic convent, protected by the nuns during wartime but treated as an outsider by the French state once the war had ended. Gille had spent many years working as an editor and a translator of other people's work; her own books revealed her to be a supremely talented writer in her own right, artfully blending the creative with the factual to produce timeless explorations of the personal nature, and social consequences, of agony.

Gille's other book was not about the Holocaust, addressing instead a different kind of trauma. *Le Crabe sur la Banquette Arrière* – or *The Crab in the Backseat*—was published in 1994, and describes the author's experiences of an illness that would eventually take her life. In a reference to the signs of the zodiac, the 'crab' in the book's title refers to cancer. The text, written in dialogue form, is a bittersweet account of the daily life of a cancer patient, using morbid humour to depict the reactions of other people (Hoerni 2016; Verghese 2020).

In one scene, a police officer pulls her over for ignoring the continuous white lines on the motorway. Élisabeth points to the X-rays in the back

[20] For a recent edition, see: Gille, É. (1994). *Le crabe sur la banquette arrière.* Paris: Mercure de France.

seat. "You're free to go", the traffic cop sheepishly responds, choosing not to enforce the law lest he be required to discuss the gory medical details. Grave illnesses can have their benefits.

Gille finds humour in the mixed messages she receives from the panoply of medical specialists she encounters. The cancer specialist: "There is a little something here and there. Just go back to your radiologist." The radiologist: "What is your cancer specialist on about? He sees cancer everywhere. You just have inflamed bronchi…" The pulmonologist: "There is nothing wrong with you, nothing at all…not a single suspicious cell." The surgeon: "…cancer, of course."

Gille phones around to get advice from friends and family. One caller tells her, "I knew it. You look awful…", while another caller concurs: "I told you you smoke far too much." Another offers words of comfort: "Well, I hope you don't let it get to you too much. A little incision, chemotherapy, and nowadays you barely even lose hair they say, radiotherapy for a while and then you'll be like new again." Someone else suggests availing of professional influence: "Don't worry, I have a specialist's number somewhere in my diary. He performs miracles. If you mention my name, you'll have an appointment within three months." But another recommends scepticism: "What kind of nonsense is that? I told you to go see my psychotherapist" (Cuthbert et al. 2019).

Gille recounts a surreal and disconnected discourse, full of compartmentalisation, self-distraction, and cognitive dissonance. A ward nurse asks her what buttock she would like to be injected in, as though she would actually have a preference. A visitor tells her she is looking well—"Healthy, with a nice colour on your cheeks"—even though she is undergoing chemotherapy and radiotherapy. Her daughter's response to her deteriorating health is to redirect her phone to Élisabeth's number, so that her mother can fend off all the boys who have been pestering her for dates: "…if it's Simon, just make something up, like I need to take you to the hospital or something."

Thematically, Gille's writings are connected by their examination of some similar themes. The Holocaust and cancer are quite different traumas, but both produce similar pressures by forcing people to think about their own—and others'—existential annihilation. Surviving, even temporarily, comes at a cost. The predicament of a cancer patient can be similar to that of a Jewish person who has lived through the Holocaust: to other people, they are living reminders of death. Bystanders are made uncomfortable by their persisting mental anguish. As Gille discovers when she gets cancer, other people find her mere presence somewhat ambiguous. They become uneasy when she is around. They feel "she should be either cured or dead."

In their own way, each of Gille's three books examines how trauma leaves a lasting influence on a wide variety of people. Victims carry heavy burdens, while others engage in mental distractions in order to get on with their lives (Miranda et al. 2025).

3.21 *C: Because Cowards Get Cancer Too*[21]—John Diamond

It's always the same: vague complaints are ignored at first, then attributed to fatigue; a loved one insists on a medical opinion; a diagnostic examination causes the doctor some concern; test results come back; cancer is diagnosed like a hammer blow; further examinations are called for; then more invasive investigations; then treatment; then more invasive treatment…

And yet it's never the same: tumours produce differing responses in different patients; everyone is unique; everyone is ill in their own way.

John Diamond (1953–2001) was a 45-year-old journalist at the BBC when he first noticed a swelling in his neck. As he recounts in his book *C: Because Cowards Get Cancer Too*, he had always felt that hypochondria was a reasonable response to any physical abnormality. After all, the sheer number of plausible pathologies produced "overwhelming statistical possibilities" (p. 17). As such he does not hesitate before consulting a doctor. The physician diagnoses glandular fever and then, after a few months with the gland in his neck still swollen, the diagnosis evolves to "persistent" glandular fever. "That's glandular fever for you," the doctor tells

[21] For a recent edition, see: Diamond, J. (1999). *C: Because Cowards Get Cancer Too*. London: Penguin.

him. A month later, his illness became "chronic" glandular fever, *chronic* being presumably more persistent than persistence itself.

Eventually, his doctor refers Diamond for more intensive assessment. Laboratory examinations, a CT scan, and a referral to an academic medical centre follow. The first thundercloud becomes visible. The surgeon removes the swelling in the neck; it is the size of a mandarin. Back at work, a sound engineer in the BBC studio teases him about his voice, and the make-up department attempt to camouflage the wound on his neck.

The cytologist finds cancer cells in the mandarin. The doctor tells the author, by phone, that he has terminal cancer, while he is watching television with his wife, Nigella. After several minutes thinking about how he felt—"I wasn't terrified at all: faced with death I was, rather, sad, angry, irritated, apologetic" (p. 37)—and while still following the plot of the episode of *EastEnders* they were watching, he eventually turns to Nigella and says: "I've got cancer." He then apologises to her. This was as much as he could explain. He didn't have any symptoms. "I didn't feel as if I were dying," he recalls.

And yet the serenity of his reaction does not result from calmness. It is the author's automatic physical response to catastrophe. "It was as involuntary a response as the scream would have been," he remarks.

Diamond determines that he is not going to panic. Sadness, that is his first reaction. He feels that undergoing cancer treatment is like joining the AA: as an alcoholic is always an alcoholic, even when not drinking, a cancer patient is always a cancer patient, even if treatment leaves them in remission.

Soon the merry-go-round starts turning. The NHS staff impress him with their dedication and empathy. Diamond discovers the phenomenon of "gradual disclosure", applied by all with whom he comes into contact: never tell the patient more than what they have found out themselves, and only give them the optimistic scenario.

Radiotherapy is especially difficult. Diamond seeks to haggle his way to a reduction: "If 30 sessions of radiotherapy can fix me, I told one of the radiotherapists, then so can 27 or 28" (p. 125). But no, they respond, the dose they give is the absolute minimum necessary, anything less and it would all be for nothing. Afterwards, the patient feels a lump in his throat which is removed in surgery ("a fairly routine operation to cut a bit out of me") and things go smoothly enough, until a tumour is found on the base of his tongue. A cancer patient is always a cancer patient. Significant intervention—the total removal of his tongue and larynx—is called for.

Diamond describes in horrible detail how difficult eating, swallowing, drinking, talking, and breathing become. Eating is like swallowing "rancid wallpaper paste", and he is tormented by the memory of what his food used to taste like. Fatigue permeates his existence. Tracheostomy care is not only complex and painful but is also distasteful for the writer and for those around him. Speech lessons help a little, but not very much. At a party to celebrate his wife's new book, he can communicate with guests only by using a pad and pencil.

Wanting to look the beast in the eye, Diamond asks his pathologist to let him peer through the microscope at the various coupes of his cancer. He develops a fascination with seeing his own cancer, and returns to the histopathology lab some weeks later for another session "to have a look at the tumour proper." He finds these samples more difficult to view, imagining how they were scraped from his throat using a scalpel "by a man with his hand in my mouth" (p. 216) (Kharade et al. 2018; Richardson et al. 2019).

Diamond is notably forthright when it comes to the science of his illness. As with other writers, he is infuriated by romanticised clichés that depict patients who 'battle' (or even 'conquer') cancer. He is especially appalled by cancer-oriented pseudoscience, and would later begin to write a book on alternative medicine (which, although unfinished, was published posthumously under the title *Snake Oil and Other Preoccupations;* Lawson 2001).

But scientific medicine is not beyond his criticism. He complains that scientists are too focused on the molecular underpinnings of illness and insufficiently consider the impact of disease on patients. He could "sift through a million pages of high-level science and learn the most intimate details of the mating habits of the squamous cell carcinoma," he records, "But none of these would tell me quickly what I needed to know, which was how would cancer affect me…" (p. 9; Tundealao et al. 2025).

He died in 2001, aged 47. On the day he passed away, the computer in his study was left switched on when he was rushed to hospital. His family discovered his final written words on-screen later that evening.

"Let me explain," Diamond had written at the end of his last unfinished paragraph (Lawson 2001).

A well-known journalist who wrote a popular weekly column for the *Sunday Times*, Diamond was certainly a masterful explainer. His accounts of his own health experiences did much to remove the social stigma around cancer in the United Kingdom, and to enhance readers' willingness to discuss the illness forthrightly (Camidge 2001; Hutchinson 2001). His very public death helped to destigmatise and demystify cancer and to promote evidence-based approaches to medicine, but without ever losing sight of the humanity at its core and the emotional pain that is at stake.

3.22 *Sickness Work*[22]—Gerhard Nijhof

Social scientists specialise in the study of other people. Only a few remember that their theories can just as easily be applied to social scientists themselves. Still fewer ever find themselves in precisely the place where their research subjects usually are. *Sickness Work* is an example of this type of reflexivity. It is the personal memoir of a professor of medical sociology—an academic who spent his career investigating the experiences of (other) people in healthcare settings—who himself finally fell seriously ill with colon carcinoma.

Gerhard Nijhof (1938–2025), a retired professor at the University of Amsterdam, knew that autobiographical texts usually make for controversial scholarship. The subjectivity of an autobiography was supposed to make it too personal, too sentimental, somewhat anecdotal, insufficiently abstracting, atheoretical, and scholarly unstructured. But he also knew that outside observers will always struggle to make sense of other people's personal narratives. He, now, could use his professional training to make sense of his own.

One of his major conclusions was that living through this type of personal experience had a profound effect on him as an academic. After a

[22] For a recent edition, see: Nijhof, G. (2018). *Sickness Work: Personal Reflections of a Sociologist.* Singapore: Palgrave Macmillan.

long career as a distinguished sociologist, cancer had now "changed [his] vision of medical sociology" (p. 1).

He came to realise that having cancer made him less judgmental of medical science. While sociologists tend to be suspicious of technology, fearing the creep of control and dependency, Nijhof found himself terrified when he was disconnected from the life-sustaining apparatus of the Intensive Care Unit. The realisation that an ordinary person like him would be so welcoming of mechanised healthcare is "very different from what I had been reading with regard to medical technology from my sociology colleagues." Sociologists "are often moralists," he observed. Cancer patients, on the other hand, develop "technological peace of mind" (p. 21).

The disruption caused by the cancer did away with his naivety. Everyday tasks suddenly required huge amounts of additional effort. He was in a hurry, as articles he was writing must now be finished quickly. Time became a precious commodity. He was constantly tired. His doctor calls it "idiopathic fatigue," explaining that surgery had left the academic with a "smaller gas tank" whose "warning light" also malfunctions (p. 18). The metaphor made sense to the doctor—an 'other' person—but was less satisfying for the patient. For Nijhof, this was an unimaginable type of fatigue that was difficult to put into words. He thought he would never be free of tiredness again. Reflecting on the challenge for sociologists of writing about this type of fatigue, given that it occurs, somewhat privately, in *other people*, he referred to it as "the puzzle of fatigue" (p. 15).

Sociologists, Nijhof noted, "focus mostly on spoken words" (p. 81). But having cancer soon revealed to him that people who are sick (or otherwise traumatised) typically regulate their thoughts using silence instead of speech. This creates a fundamental problem for social scientists. The testimony underlying much of their work becomes skewed: a talkative minority will likely receive disproportionate airtime. For Nijhof, this required a fundamental change of approach for sociologists. Sociologists, he argues, "should listen more to the silence" (p. 81).

Nijhof structured his thoughts as an academic would, packaging them into seven chapters with high-level conceptual titles: *Disruption*; *Incantation*; *Collective Disruption*; *Sickness Work*; *Control*; *The Outside World*; and *Legitimation*. Ever sobre, he focused on navigating the human foibles he encounters when living with his illness: caring for his stoma, eating in restaurants, giving lectures, visiting friends, planning a holiday. "I had been working on illness as a medical sociologist for thirty years, but I had never been ill," he reflected. But now, "it was suddenly different. I had cancer."

"Hospital beds are single beds," he recorded, but being sick is a collective disruption. Nijhof felt that medical sociology, while acknowledging social contexts more than most academic disciplines, remains almost as individualising as medicine. The social intricacies of illness continue to be underexplored. Medical sociologists usually say that sickness leads to "network shrinkage," the gradual loss of social contact over time. But Nijhof felt this overlooks the fact that close relationships usually intensify. Not only that, but new and energising interdependencies emerge. The sick person relies on others, but others too come to rely on them (Samuel et al. 2022). Caregiving for a loved one is not an 'occupation', it is more of a compulsion, a self-identity that must be fulfilled. "Illness does something to relationships," Nijhof argued, "but what exactly does it do?" (p. 41). For Nijhof, sociology had little to say on the nature of love in illness, because "people are not eager to discuss it" (p. 41). Yet again, he felt, sociologists should pay attention to the silences they encounter.

Nijhof suggested that the way other people react to a sick person frequently reveals the gap between the observer and the observed. Nijhof himself would become angry at well-intentioned remarks that suggested his illness was being taken away from him. Being told that he was "looking well" would negate his status as an ill person and deny him the privileges of the sick. "Disqualified, that's how I sometimes felt," he recalled. "Silenced" (p. 93). For him, such cheerfulness served as a signal that the patient should stop identifying with their illness and rejoin the world of the healthy. It communicated a kind of repudiation, the compliment a cover for a deeper message: "don't bother me with your illness" (p. 94).

Nijhof noted that much of this thinking is unconscious, that illness is "socially regulated" in ways that make things more comfortable for the well majority. Nobody would ever admit to deliberately marginalising the medically stricken; in fact, "they would be outraged to be accused of such a thing" (p. 94). And yet it happens all the time. "Frequently," Nijhof concluded, "the sick just let it pass" (p. 94; Eklund et al. 2025).

Sickness Work succeeds in being dispassionate, as the standards of academic scholarship demand. Its sobre conclusions are somewhat echoed by emerging empirical research into patients' perceptions of treatment goals (El-Jawari et al. 2020), patient-physician relationships (Samuel et al. 2022), and so-called life review therapy (Kleijn et al. 2021).

By the end of the book, Nijhof was on the road to recovery and then to work. He had no idea what is still possible and what might no longer be possible. The sick have to explore, he felt, be curious, and experiment. He observed how doctors seem to think of patients mainly as lying on a table or in a bed. But being ill is a time-consuming and overwhelming set of activities. Patients have to discover a lot about themselves, and reorganise the logistics of their day-to-day lives. This is the "sickness work" that Nijhof referenced in the title of his book.

For Nijhof, social scientists too have much sickness work to do.

3.23 *The Undying*[23]—Anne Boyer

For some autobiographical writers, using the words "I" and "cancer" in the same sentence is almost taboo. As the American poet and essayist Anne Boyer (1973–) points out in her own 2019 cancer memoir, *The Undying*, "'I' is sometimes annihilated by cancer, but sometimes preemptively annihilated by the person it represents…" (p. 5). But she is not one of those authors. Instead, she highlights the following statement as especially significant: "I was diagnosed with breast cancer in 2014, at the age of forty-one" (p. 9). This statement, she suggests, is more than merely factual. It is *ideological.*

Boyer is clear: she is going to talk about cancer as a cultural fact. Like many writers in her situation, she rejects the culturally prevalent narrative of brave patients battling against the odds for their own survival. This narrative, she suggests, amounts to a form of victim-blaming. By casting cancer patients as the prime agents of their own welfare, individuals are implied to be responsible for *everything* that happens to them. They are

[23] For a recent edition, see: Boyer, A. (2020). *The Undying: A Meditation on Modern Illness*. London: Penguin.

therefore their *own* problem, not *society's* problem. The powers-that-be can rest easy when the source of human suffering is located in individuals. For Boyer, this narrative of cancer as a *battle fought by patients* is little more than a political message, a promotion of "neoliberal self-management" (p. 9), with everything from mammograms to "green smoothies" on offer to distract the sick from, say, societal injustice and health inequalities.

The very idea of surviving, Boyer explains, is an inherently one-sided concept, where only the underdog is rooted for. Those who fail to survive are downgraded. Boyer describes this ideology of the *survivor* as akin to "a betrayal of the dead" (p. 290). She recoils at the use of pink ribbons to signify survivorship, and at the hysteria of declaring breast cancer, in particular, to be such a "hot" charity cause.

Many international readers will be perturbed by Boyer's descriptions of medicine in the United States. What is likely framed in terms of individual choice and convenience for Americans can seem utterly disempowering and belittling from a distance. Boyer explains that nearly half of American mastectomies are now performed on an out-patient basis: despite the anaesthesia, the cutting, the bleeding, and (not least) the life-changing physical alterations, patients are not even afforded a bed in which to recover overnight. Such procedures, Boyer explains, are now commonly referred to as "drive-by mastectomies" (p. 155).

Boyer sees a tumour—her own—for the first time in her life, on a computer screen. What she previously only read about ("The unholy granite substance in my breast", she recalls Alice James having written in 1892), she could now see for herself, "round with a long craggy finger jutting from it" (p. 13). There is no looking away. And yet, as merely the patient, she must photograph the tumour with her iPhone in order to possess the picture for herself.

As the investigations continue, the diagnostic machinery takes over: the "detectors with names made of letters" (MRI, CT, PET), the heavy-duty medical earmuffs, the "cinematic beeps" emanating from esoteric devices (which include, intriguingly, a "wand"). "Radiology," Boyer muses, "turns a person made of feelings and flesh into a patient made of lights and shadows" (p. 15). But whatever the machinery clarifies to the professionals does not always have meaning for the patients. "They tell me I have cancer," whispers the man next to her in the oncology waiting room, "but I have my doubts" (p. 18).

With algorithmic banality, her surgeon explains that "the greatest risk factor for breast cancer was having breasts" (p. 29). Strictly speaking, this is true, of course, but such approaches do little to nullify the complaint some patients have that their doctors treat them 'like numbers'. Procedural guidelines prevent the surgeon from explaining the biopsy results because Boyer has arrived at the clinic unaccompanied. The rules say that somebody else must be with her at this moment. Boyer's friend Cara dutifully drives across town so that the diagnosis can be revealed. She must do this on her lunch break because only family members are legally facilitated to leave work for such reasons. In the United States, Boyer explains, "If you are loved outside the enclosure of family, the law doesn't care how deeply…" (p. 29). With all the personnel prerequisites now met, the surgeon can announce "what we already knew", namely, that Boyer has at least one cancerous tumour in her left breast. Cara can go back to work.

Later Boyer receives a glossy brochure, entitled *Your Oncology Journey*, complete with a smiling silver-haired woman on its cover. It is difficult to tell whether it is medical advice or some kind of marketing campaign. The positives are certainly accentuated, but Boyer feels she has little to smile about. The diagnosis is ominous: "Triple Negative" breast cancer, for which there is no targeted treatment (Turkman et al. 2016).

Without much ostentation, it is decided that the doctors will "take [Boyer's] breasts and discard them in an incinerator" (p. 37). Feeling like a product on an assembly line, Boyer's anger and disappointment run deep. It is another example of how "the boundaries of our bodies" become broken by the system. "Everything we were supposed to keep inside of us now seems to fall out," Boyer points laments. "Blood from chemotherapy-induced nosebleeds drips on the sheets, the paperwork, the CVS receipts, the library books. We can't stop crying. We emit foul odors. We throw up. We have poisonous vaginas and poisoned sperm. Our urine is so toxic that the signs in the bathroom instruct patients to flush twice. We do not look like people: we look like people with cancer. We resemble a disease before we resemble ourselves" (p. 49).

Boyer's critique continues. American healthcare, she argues—even *cancer* care—is focused primarily on producing profitable treatments, not on helping people get better. Insurance companies, hospital organisations, and pharmaceutical companies are the main players. *The Undying* is more than just a memoir; its subtitle casts it as "a meditation on modern illness."

The contrast between Boyer's account and the idealised science of medical journal articles is stark. Even so-called multidisciplinary care approaches (e.g., Bellon et al. 2020) appear heavily technocratic and logistical. The human experience of cancer, including triple-negative breast cancer, is frequently written about by doctors (McNeil 2018; Post et al. 2025; Swain 2017; Turkman et al. 2016), but the broader psychosocial view is often curtailed. Even psychologists focus mostly on perceptions and relationships in the immediate personal context, rather than on the economic, cultural, and political realities in which cancer patients are enmeshed.

Sick or not sick, dying or undying, the citizens will always be dragged back to their place in society. Ten days after her surgery, Boyer returns to work.

3.24 *Poems About Cancer*[24]—Hans Lodeizen

As evidenced on these pages, many writers, across many literary genres, have creatively touched upon the theme of physical illness, their combined endeavours resulting in a new branch of academic scholarship, often labelled 'Lit Med' (for 'literature + medicine'). Nobel literary nominee Simon Vestdijk was one of its pioneers, writing an academic treatise on 'the ill person in novels' some six decades ago (Vestdijk 1964). Interest has broadened as well as deepened in succeeding years. Nowadays, a plethora of books, as well as other academic publications, explore the use of art, painting, film, and even music, as lenses through which the human experience of illness, and specifically that of cancer, can be viewed (Kaptein et al. 2018). The arts have become so salient in medical discourse that specialist journals, such as *Psycho-Oncology* and *Supportive*

[24] For a recent publication of Lodeizen's collected poetry, see: Lodeizen, H. (2007). *Verzameide Gedichten*. Amsterdam: G. A. von Oorschot.

Care in Cancer, frequently present the creative arts as a medically essential dimension of human existence, one central to helping patients succeed at 'living with' their illness.

However, within the panoply of crafts usually showcased in this regard, poetry is something of a niche pursuit. Poems about cancer can be difficult to find (although, ironically, the acronym 'POEM' crops up relatively frequently in medical literature searches, having been used to denote 'patient-oriented evidence that matters'; e.g., Slawson and Shaughnessy 1997).

By far the best book on poetry regarding cancer is *Cancer Poetry* by Iain Twiddy (2015). Two interesting collections of poetry concerning illness more generally—*Mijn dokter is een goede dokter [My doctor is a good doctor]*, edited by G. J. Bremer and Wim Hazeu, which appeared in 1974, and Michael Salcman's 2015 anthology, *Poetry in Medicine*—each contain a selection of works dealing with cancer. The former features two poems by the influential Dutch poet, Hans Lodeizen (1924–1950).

Lodeizen lived a life characterised by various forms of solitude. Raised in a wealthy district, with a cold and distant father, the young Lodeizen became a fearful child, who struggled to handle the rough manners of his peers (Hilberdink 2007). At one point he failed his high school examinations and temporarily ran away from home. Later, while at university, he left his law degree in Leiden to study biology in the United States, eventually dropping out of his American college and returning to the Netherlands. His desire to write poetry clashed with his father's plan that he run the family business. His sexuality clashed with society's conservatism, and at the age of 24 he was arrested for having sex with a male lover. Shortly afterwards he developed leukaemia. Within two years he had died.

In the midst of his illness, Lodeizen muses about the future. "I am 25 years old and my life is just beginning," he writes. "But no, it was later than he thought…For though the calendar said, behold, the spring is here/He felt his heart falling out like a dead flower". When these words are read in class to first-year medical students, the young trainees often become uneasy. "But isn't leukaemia very treatable?" is a very common query. "Not always," will be the unfortunately grim response (Niscola et al. 2025).

Lodeizen's verse also sheds light on the impact of doctor–patient communication. In a poem entitled "When you are sad", he observes: "When you are sad, the doctor says/You need to eat more…that's logical." But however logical the advice may be, as far as Lodeizen is concerned "the doctor does not think about me." Yet again, the young Lodeizen finds himself alone. Too frequently, medical attention focuses more on science than on subjectivity.

In 1971, Bremer read these words at a public lecture to commemorate his appointment as lecturer at the medical faculty of Leiden University (Bremer and Hazeu 1972). In his remarks, Bremer highlighted the way in which Lodeizen's poem toys with this question of perspectives. Can patients and doctors ever see things the same way? The power of poetry, he argued, is to help bridge these inherent gaps.

Solitude need not be perennial.

3.25 *Black Rain*[25]—Masuji Ibuse

All human bodies reflect a universal genetic template: familiar shapes duplicated from person to person; flesh and physiology copied-and-pasted onto a recurring musculoskeletal frame. Human beings share a single range of physical capacities, with equivalent strengths and potentials, and yet, by the same token, the same corporeal vulnerabilities. Western science too (assisted in no small way by colonialism) has become ubiquitous around the world. It is no surprise therefore that medical oncologists from different nations can readily understand one another. Regardless of where such physicians have been trained, they find it easy to discuss cancer's biological processes and the treatments that might be used to target them.

Every year, physicians meet at the same international conferences. They read the same articles in the same journals. When it comes to medicine, they speak the same scientific language. Or at least they do until concepts such as 'quality of life', 'patient-reported outcomes', or 'symptom perceptions' are discussed. When the conversation turns to

[25] For a recent edition, see: Ibuse, M. (2012). Black Rain. Tokyo: Kodansha International.

psychological experiences of cancer, it suddenly becomes clear that there are, in fact, many separate worlds (Dein 2004; Kaptein et al. 2011, 2013).

This is because human experience is something that is *perceived* rather than scientifically encoded. Human experience is, after all, *experienced* by the *human*. An oncologist will be able to predict what a particular chemotherapy will do to a patient's red blood cell count, but they will be unable to predict the person's exact fears about what cancer means for their lives, their livelihoods, or their relationships. What constitutes an acceptable intensity or type of 'side-effect' is often unique to the individual concerned. The traumas and choices precipitated by cancer are emotionally *personal* ones.

Psychologists have long pointed out that even the basics of medical treatment are reliant on a patient's perception of what is going on. Even the most sophisticated drug therapies will prove pretty useless if a patient fails to adhere to them. A patient may simply not comply with their doctor's instructions to take this particular medication according to that particular schedule. They may feel instead that the exactness of timings and dosages doesn't really matter. Or they may feel their illness is incurable and so there is no point in taking tablets. Or they may feel that their illness will in fact *cure itself* if given enough time. Or they may simply feel *tired* of all this medical intrusion and want now to prioritise other aspects of their existence. Simply put, because modern medicine relies so much on patient cooperation, how a patient *feels* about their illness will be a key determinant of how their treatment—and thus their illness—actually ends up proceeding.

Of course, perceptions and experiences vary from place to place, which is why conversations among international oncologists often go awry when they start discussing psychological factors. Living in a particular locale will imbue a person with particular perceptions and attitudes, compiled and shared across decades of particular events. In some instances, collective traumas experienced generations ago will end up shaping cultural attitudes in ways that leave their imprint decades later. One's attitude to life-threatening illness will, at least in part, be filtered through the life-and-death attitudes that one derives from one's cultural surroundings.

In his 1965 novel *Black Rain*, the Japanese author Masuji Ibuse (1898–1993) subtly interweaves cultural and social factors into his account of one such collective trauma and the outpouring of cancer that was left in its wake.

Ibuse was born in a village in Hiroshima Prefecture, Japan, in 1898. He studied French and art history in Tokyo and worked as a war correspondent in Singapore. In his forties, he found himself back home in Hiroshima on August 6, 1945, the day an atomic bomb was dropped on the city, destroying two-thirds of its buildings and killing over a hundred thousand of its civilians. It was the first use of a nuclear weapon in armed conflict.

On the ground, the traumatised survivors, surrounded by crushed buildings and horrific casualties, were unsure of what precisely had happened. Many felt that several bombs had been dropped on them, rather than just one. A few hours after the attack, as described by Ibuse, black rain begins to fall from the sky. The raindrops are the size of marbles. Some people speculate about "a new weapon" that caused all this, but others believe an "oil bomb" or a "gas bomb" has been used (p. 35). With apparently uninjured people beginning to fall sick and die later that day, others fear they have been attacked with a "poison bomb" or a form of tear gas, or with some other device that released "dysentery germs" or "bacteria" (p. 200). It is only after a few days that the word "atomic bomb" starts to circulate. The mystery of what triggered the catastrophe must have contributed to a feeling of ultimate alienation.

Black rain continues to fall from the jellyfish-shaped cloud, a spectre that hangs over the city for days before slowly descending onto the earth. Soap and water do not remove the black rain from people's bodies. Trying to rub it off with a cloth leads to peeling skin and horrific infections.

Black Rain is a documentary novel. Ibuse weaves in eyewitness accounts, personal diaries, and official reports. He tells how rescue teams, after arriving in Hiroshima, recorded seeing victims with humanly unrecognisable faces the size of watermelons, with burnt hair and eyelids fused closed. Survivors cannot even recognise their own close friends or family members. The aid workers try to write names in ink on people's skin, as if tagging stray farm animals. A doctor describes the backs of the survivors: "red and lumpy like a turkey's comb, and the skin had come off like a sheet of oiled paper...the intense heat had numbed the nerves under the burnt skin so that no pain was felt" (p. 118). Emergency responders find themselves trapped in a stench-ridden hell: thousands of corpses burning in the open air; wretched survivors in terrible pain, soon to be overwhelmed by hunger and thirst.

Ibuse's descriptions in *Black Rain* cast survivors' psychological responses as almost reserved and unemotional. A woman who has not heard from her brother is calmly resigned to the fact that he is probably dead by now. There is hardly any crying or yelling. People are just numb, or at least silent, perhaps influenced by the Japanese taboo against bothering others with your problems.

The inhabitants of Hiroshima continue to get ill: fever, diarrhoea, abscesses, white skin, hair loss, broken teeth, pain, mud-coloured nails; sedimentation rates are abnormal, too many white blood cells and too few red ones. The Emperor of Japan announces his country's surrender over a radio broadcast, the first time everyone hears his voice.

The novel switches back and forth from August 1945 to a period many years later, when lead character Shizuma Shigematsu becomes the legal guardian of his niece, Yasuko. He encounters persistent difficulty finding a suitable husband for his niece, who is widely believed to have been contaminated by the infamous 'black rain'. Ultimately, the rumours prove true. Despite Shizuma's hopes to the contrary, and even though many years have passed, Yasuko eventually falls ill with cancer. Another victim of the ravages of Hiroshima's nuclear cataclysm.

Fifty years after Ibuse's novel was published, a Japanese judge ruled that citizens living outside the worst-affected parts of the city should be entitled to free medical care to treat the late effects of radiation exposure (McCurry 2015). Over time it has emerged that even the 'hibakusha' (bomb survivors; see Naono 2019; Terayama et al. 2021) were contaminated by radiation, and so deserve some protection, albeit belated, from the terrible black rain.

3.26 *The Wounded Storyteller*[26]—Arthur W. Frank

The Canadian sociologist Arthur W. Frank (1946–) was once banned from putting up posters advertising a support meeting organised by patients in a cancer centre. That was in 1990. Some 30 years later, it is now difficult to avoid such posters in public spaces, especially on the notice boards of healthcare facilities. Patient empowerment and self-advocacy have become 'negotiable', spawning a guild whose members are marked by emblems such as pink (and other coloured) lapel ribbons. Nonetheless, as Frank argues, public discussion of cancer remains problematic. Restrictions are applied. We can by all means speak publicly about cancer, but only within approved frames of reference. Frank's 1995 book, beautifully titled *The Wounded Storyteller*, explores the exacting parameters of this discourse.

Frank has observed and listened closely to many patients with cancer as well as to their physicians. He is also an expert by experience, having lived not only through myocardial infarction but also testicular carcinoma. He notes, to his dismay, that his many medical files contain only the physician's accounts of his illnesses. They say nothing about his own personal experiences of them. His 'narratives', he notes—along with the narratives of patients in general—remain officially off the record (Bayliss 1998; Cassell 2004; Frank 1991; Hunsaker 1999; Miller et al. 2025).

In *The Wounded Storyteller*, Frank focuses on storytelling as a feature of 'postmodern' medicine. In postmodern medicine, he argues, personal perspectives dominate what society considers to be valid information. As such, postmodern medicine stands in contrast to (and has largely supplanted) the older 'modern' medicine, where for decades science and technology were believed to hold the key to explaining how people become sick and/or well.

Frank suggests that patients' storytelling narratives emerge in three permissible forms. These are the narratives that communities tend to gravitate towards, the storyboards and plotlines that societal and personal

[26] For a recent edition, see: Frank, A. (2013). *The Wounded Storyteller: Body, Illness, and Ethics*, Second Edition. Chicago: University of Chicago Press.

preferences end up favouring. Individuals—but also institutions—find it easier to draw on familiar templates when crafting explanations of patients' lives. According to Frank, shared narratives can be helpful, by assisting patients to shape their own stories in coherent and meaningful ways. But culturally shared narratives can also be a hindrance. The inclination to fall back on readymade narratives can serve to limit the understanding of those who *listen* to patients' stories, driving them to interpret patient accounts as only ever having a limited range of possible meanings. Novel and unique experiences end up not being heard.

The first narrative that Frank outlines is that of *restitution*. This occurs when a patient is suddenly laid low but then recovers fully from their illness. In the restitution narrative, illness is a temporary disruption, most likely addressable by medical intervention. The restitution narrative is viewed very favourably by patients, practitioners, hospital directors, and health insurers—not to mention also by government officials and the producers of television drug commercials—essentially, by any audience that is gratified by the prospect of problems being rapidly resolved.

Frank describes how restitution narratives can be framed retrospectively, but also prospectively. Patients can obsess over stories of recovery even before they have actually happened. In fact, the persistent focus on future recovery is often a mainstay of cancer support groups. Patients are encouraged to view their future lives in remission as inevitable and assured. For Frank, this type of narrative has a clear downside, in that not all patients actually recover. He describes attending a cancer support group in which a patient who broke down in tears in despair at their worsening health was ignored by the other group members. "Thus the group expressed its preference for restitution stories," Frank observed, "and its discomfort at hearing illness told in other narratives" (p. 78).

Frank's second narrative is that of *chaos*. In many respects, the chaos narrative is the opposite of the restitution narrative: "its plot imagines life never getting better" (p. 97). The patient's story has no logical order, no timeline, no perspective on change, and no medical improvement. The patient will describe having no influence over their illness; terrifyingly, they will often state that their care providers have also lost control. The familiar question "Why me?" encapsulates the despair of the chaos narrative. Patients find themselves trapped in an everlasting present, overwhelmed by dismay and unable to reflect on their lives. The chaos narrative is an incessant doom spiral. Newly encountered adverse experiences are not approached in isolation, because they trigger the patients' memories of all the other adversities they have experienced. Chaos narratives can be especially difficult for patients to escape, or for their loved ones to listen to.

The third of Frank's narratives is the *quest narrative*. In this narrative, a patient may not feel that recovery is assured, but they are also not overwhelmed by the prospect of open-ended illness. They look suffering straight in the face, perhaps seeing it as a valuable life lesson. "The quest," Frank explains, "is defined by the ill person's belief that something is to be gained through the experience" (p. 115).

In the restitution narrative, the outcome is determined by the medical intervention; in the chaos narrative, there is no coherent outcome at all. But the quest narrative positions patients as the protagonists of their own exploits. In the quest narrative, the outcome is steered by the patient themselves, and so "only in quest stories does the *teller* have a story to tell" (p. 115). By taking control of their narrative, the patient "holds chaos at bay" (p. 115).

For Frank, even though the quest narrative has no guaranteed ending, it represents a lucrative form of storytelling. It assists patients to feel that they are more important than their own illness, instead of being defined by it. It facilitates their adjustment to symptoms and to treatment side effects and improves their relationships with healthcare providers. Quest narratives are often positively contagious, helping to show fellow patients a way to escape from chaos narratives. Despite all this, according to Frank, the quest narrative is frequently resisted. Patients themselves often react lukewarmly to physical therapists, social workers, or psychologists when they encourage them to focus on 'living with' cancer. But once a physician starts to speak about new drugs or treatments for cancer, the restitution narrative takes over very quickly.

Frank points out that contemporary cancer discourse most often reverts to a narrative of restitution. Patients are trained to refer to themselves as "cancer survivors", even before they are fully in remission. The title of one academic journal—the *Journal of Cancer Survivorship*—imposes this norm quite starkly.

The restitution narrative can also be detected when healthcare trainees explain their occupational motivations. Only a few trainees express an interest in devoting themselves to conducting medical research; by far the majority are committed to 'helping people' (as though medical research is of no help to anyone; Hughes 2018). But even where research is contemplated, only some of it is recognised as counting; most charities and research funding agencies prioritise the 'search for a cure' over other types of empirical investigation.

The bias towards restitution also affects what scholarship gets published. Peer reviewers of manuscripts will object to papers that focus on the experiences of the terminally ill, encouraging authors to balance their writing with reference to patients who recover ("These days, cancer is treatable!" is a common refrain).

As Frank points out, it is as though those who are about to die are undeserving of their own narrative.

3.27 *The Following Scan Will Last Five Minutes*[27]—Lieke Marsman

This brief book by the Dutch poet Lieke Marsman (1990–) is very approachable (as is its English-language edition, translated by the Dutch-British poet Sophie Collins). However, it takes a little longer to read than the five-minute scan mentioned in its title. *The Following Scan Will Last Five Minutes* (published in Dutch in 2018 and in English in 2019) contains a selection of short poems, interposed by a reflective essay in which the author describes the time she was first diagnosed with cancer.

The essay explains how the author, then 27 years old, was sent for a scan after she herself, along with a coterie of healthcare personnel—two physiotherapists, a general practitioner, an orthopaedic surgeon, a radiologist, and a neurologist, no less—all suspected that she was suffering from burnout. The test result reveals otherwise: a chondrosarcoma of 80 × 90 × 100 millimetres was found in her upper back. Whether in Dutch

[27] For a recent edition, see: Marsman, L. (2019). *The Following Scan Will Last Five Minutes* (translated by Sophie Collins). Liverpool: Pavilion Poetry.

('*chondrosarcoom*') or in English, the word *chondrosarcoma* is inherently sonorous, implicitly singing its appeal to any poet. Marsman persistently weaves the baroque with the banal, writing in one of her poems: "For years you have no doubt/been googling every freckle. Just recently/you were at the doctor's with a patch/of dry skin on your leg/Diagnosis: too much shower gel/But on hearing the word *chondrosarcoma*/you went home and immediately unplugged your router…"

A poet's voice can help shine light on the random thoughts that intrude in moments of crisis. When Marsman views an image of her tumour, she sees "a big white ball containing lots of other, smaller white balls", which "reminds [her] of a cauliflower" (p. 23). Such a voice can be especially revealing about patients' experiences of diagnostic examinations. It is a shame that researchers cannot recruit more poets to testify about what it feels like to be examined in this way.

Evocatively, Marsman uses just four words to capture how the disembodied radiographer instructs her as she lies in the MRI machine: "The MRI tunnel speaks" (in fact, this is where she is first told that "The following scan will last five minutes"; p. 17). Events begin to unfold in her mind, as mechanistic detail mingles with metaphorical flourish: "Contrast agent/The stench of anaesthetic/A beach ball in your nose/A volleyball in your stomach" (p. 17). As she lies there in the machine, Marsman records, "Poetry fills this empty head" (p. 18; cf. Kaptein et al. 2025).

Many of the poems reflect more of these random thoughts than they do the particulars of cancer treatment. Some of the poems are exclusively based on these intrusive mid-scan ideas. In one, entitled *The Following Scan Will Last Three Minutes*, Marsman begins with the appeal, "God, grant us the confidence of a mediocre white man…" before railing against the patriarchy and capitalism ("while men initiate price wars/or regular wars/the kind involving weapons" (p. 14). Cancer is not mentioned at all.

In the essay, Marsman describes how a major surgery proves successful (insofar as "my arm is still attached"; p. 24). The author can read, write, and follow the news. Her illness story is more than an articulation of illness. The practicalities of assistance, breakdown, health insurance, and politics colour her writing. She is one of those critical patients who force doctors to do their clinical and scientific utmost. She is unfailingly grateful, but also assertive and politically aware.

Despite her own illness—or perhaps because of it—Marsman seeks to contextualise her suffering within a broader human experience. She describes how her deteriorating working memory affects her ability to do her laundry. She then imagines how this cognitive deficit would affect her if she were a refugee seeking asylum after escaping a warzone, fleeing execution and persecution by travelling to a country where bureaucrats speak a different language to you, but where those same bureaucrats will send you back to the warzone if you are unable to fill out their forms correctly. (Once again evoking the banal, she notes how in the Netherlands, asylum seekers must complete a citizenship test with questions such as "What is an acceptable way of celebrating your birthday with your co-workers?"; p. 33.) For Marsman, sloppy laundry is not the worst outcome. It is hardly worth complaining about. And she still has two arms. For now. (In fact, some years after her book was published, Marsman would indeed lose her arm to cancer.)

Marsman approaches the dilemmas that surround cancer patient sloganeering. She wonders whether it is reasonable to describe her life as a "battle with cancer" (p. 35). Might that metaphor place an undue burden of responsibility on cancer patients, pre-emptively blaming those who die for having battled insufficiently? Again, Marsman explores the issue through a better-directed comparison. No, she feels, the battle metaphor is not unfair on those who lose the fight: "What is unfair for those who died of cancer is the fact that there are others who have never been sick and yet feel they have the right to tell cancer patients how to talk about their own illness" (p. 35). In warfare, it is important to know exactly who your adversaries should be.

Marsman's account of doctor–patient interactions is also enlightening. After recovering from surgery, she reads what the doctor has written in her discharge note: "Patient was able to leave hospital in good condition." In her poet's voice, she feels this would be better rendered as something more reflective of her experienced reality. She suggests: "Patient was able to climb out of bed unsupported and no longer cries when hoisted onto ward's mobile toilet" (p. 25). The implied divide between what physicians view as important and how patients view their own priorities reveals the poet's subjective perceptiveness.

Research on life with chondrosarcoma is relatively scarce, with one Norwegian study describing how patients tend to end up in one of three statuses: 'back to normal', 'a new normal', or '[permanent] struggle' (Fauske et al. 2019). Overall quality of life remains low for these patients (Pereira et al. 2019). Partly this can result from the challenge of dealing with other people who are well. Marsman does not feel comfortable talking with other people in her life about her cancer. "Sometimes I worry that cancer has made me egotistical," she explains. "I feel ashamed. So many people get sick." And yet she feels compelled to share: "And still I have the unerring sense that my disease is deserving of constant discussion" (p. 37). Calling upon others for care is also a source of distress: "I don't want to be washed by the person with whom I share my bed at night." She feels this involves a disconcerting level of infantile regression, depriving her of her hard-earned adult joy at "not [having] to constantly call my parents for their help with this or that" (p. 36; Paulson et al. 2024).

Ultimately, Marsman adopts a contrived ambivalence towards her own suffering, an almost witty form of sarcasm. She accepts that it would be best to avoid being "foolish" or "needlessly melodramatic", but allows herself some leeway: "only a little" melodrama would be fine (p. 39).

Marsman talks of "sink[ing] away/into the morphine-sweet unreality of the everyday" (p. 7). It is a reminder that despite all the medical interventions, she is, at heart, her own person, an ordinary human being with thoughts, opinions, and desires that range far beyond her diagnosis.

The poet's voice reminds us that an illness is but one life experience, a single concern among many.

3.28 *Alien Sleepers*[28]—Verena Stefan

An "alien sleeper" (*Fremdschläfer*) is a bureaucratic term in Switzerland for an asylum seeker who is caught staying overnight at a place different from the one they have been assigned to by the authorities. The Swiss-born author Verena Stefan (1947–2017) is not the first writer to be struck by the idea that a cancerous tumour is itself an interloper within the

[28] For a recent edition, see: Stefan, V. (2007). *Fremdschläfer*. Zürich: Ammann.

human body. In her 2007 autobiographical novel *Fremdschläfer*, Stefan draws parallels between the experiences of immigration and those of illness: foreigners in a strange land, and foreign entities inside the human body (McMullin 2016).

Stefan moves to Canada for love, but feels like a stranger in her new country. When she discovers a lump in her breast—a *Fremdkörper*—her alienation becomes complete. The complexities of Stefan's displacement are encapsulated in geography and language. For example, most of the book is set in Quebec, whilst Bern, Switzerland, is Stefan's historical homeplace; French Canadian and Bern-Deutsch become her two languages.

Her female radiologist is young, well-groomed and meticulous, impressing Stefan with her style and confidence. She then immediately resorts to a more familiar and clichéd description, rendered in Canadian French: "elle est bien dans sa peau" ("she is comfortable in her own skin"; p. 23). In this way, Stefan juxtaposes the elaborateness of her personal Swiss identity with the cold second-language mundanity of her new surroundings as an immigrant. The richness of her old life is linguistically contrasted with the brutality of her new situation (Schmidt 2018).

Stefan has not only moved countries, she has migrated to the land of the sick. Her physical descriptions of breasts, breast cancer, and chemotherapy should be eye-opening for practitioners who treat breast cancer. She highlights how women have many attributes besides their medically relevant anatomies. Their personhood also involves "eroticism, pride, shame, desire, lust, comfort, nourishment, feeding, care, violence, insult, injury, competition, envy, love, break-ups, children, attractiveness, ageing, fear" (p. 24). (Notably, the breast is associated, at least obliquely, with many of these concepts.) But now she must learn to identify with new words: *lymph nodes*, *receptors*, *oncology*, and worst of all, *malignant*. The words *medicine* and *healing* are less commonly encountered. Instead, the medical messaging is much more indirect, more subtle. Stefan learns to focus on the new colours she sees at the outpatient clinic: peach pink, apricot orange, and apple green. She feels that the examination bench looks more like a gurney than a place of treatment. She is left to ruminate by herself. Are these cancer cells, those damn *Fremdkörper*, swimming through her liver, lungs, brain? Her entire body?

The diagnostic announcement, when it comes, is clear, albeit delivered in alien French: "*C'est un cancer.*" Stefan had noticed that the distance created when communicating in a second language can often be protective. This time, however, it is different. The protection has worn off. "The sentence hits right in the heart" (p. 52).

Whatever language you are speaking, once you have said the word *cancer* in your own voice, there is no going back, she concludes. The diagnosis creates new types of vigilance. In the waiting room, she now watches the other patients differently, wondering about their caps, their hats, their turbans, and their scarves, and speculating about the women who have short hair. Are these heads significant? Is that person's hair falling out or growing? How about that person? And then she realises that she herself is going to be analysed this way. Her hairstyle too will be medically profiled.

A skull-and-crossbones symbol adorns the milk-glass door of the Nuclear Medicine department. Within the machine, Stefan feels as though her body has become transparent, as if she has been placed under a magnifying glass. She reflects back to past years. When did this all start, she wonders. Did she have cancer when she was on holiday the previous summer? Or even before that? In the car park after the consultation, she describes the post-traumatic feelings of a newly diagnosed cancer patient: "…you feel overwhelmed, depressed, ill" (p. 63; Sánchez-Gómez et al. 2025).

The author takes the reader into her disconnected and alienated world, a place that is highly complex, confusingly layered, and full of symbolism. In such a place, communication is often nonverbal. She *sees* everyone else's fear. The terror in people's faces evokes many messages: the person who knows they will die; the person whose life has just been turned upside down; the person who just does not know yet whether they actually have cancer. Meanwhile, mainstream culture continues to bombard people with jarring depictions of normality. Pictures of healthy breasts, both covered and naked, can unexpectedly appear, at any time, online or in magazines. Even in newspapers. Reminders of what could have been are unavoidable.

In such a world, information is not merely spoken or seen. Communication is multisensory. Even smell is loaded with meaning. Stefan can especially tell she is sick on days before chemotherapy: "I stink…[My] urine stinks. The urine smells of something that has no name, an ashtray full of cigarette butts left in the rain and dissolved, plus a burnt smell, maybe burnt rubber" (p. 117).

Verena Stefan found herself trapped in an uncertain world where words and meaning were suspended by illness. Ultimately, illness made her travel ever further, right to the terminus, as she was to die from breast cancer a decade after she wrote *Fremdschläfer*. As Susan Sontag had proposed, illness makes migrants of us all, travellers from the kingdom of wellness to unfamiliar territories of disease: "…sooner or later each of us is obliged, at least for a spell, to identify ourselves as citizens of that other place" (Sontag 1978). The journey of Swiss-born Verena Stefan ended physically in Canada. But cancer made her an alien sleeper. She was in many different places at once, never either in one or another.

Never sure of where, or how, she belonged.

3.29 *Love Life*[29]—Ray Kluun

Like sex, drugs, or rock 'n' roll, when it comes to sensationalist plot points in fiction, cancer certainly sells. If you ask a lecture room full of medical students to name a novel that depicts living with cancer, many hands will go up. In the Netherlands, at least, one novel will certainly be cited: *Love Life*, by Ray Kluun (1964–). This fast-paced duplicitous romantic drama is certainly exciting. So marketable, in fact, that in 2009 it was made into a movie—*Komt een vrouw bij de dokter* ("A woman comes to the doctor"; although marketed more simply in English, as *Stricken*). Starring a trio of popular Dutch celebrity actors in its leading roles, the movie was the highest-grossing film in the Netherlands that year. It remains one of only six Dutch movies ever to be conferred with 'Diamond Film' status in the Netherlands, a formal award for films that sell more than one million tickets at the domestic box office.

The novel itself has been translated into several languages and has sold millions of copies worldwide. While a massive seller, it is not a work that is rated highly by literary scholars or book reviewers. Nonetheless, *Love*

[29] For a recent edition, see: Kluun, R. (2007). *Love Life: A Novel*. New York: St. Martin's Press.

Life retains a reputation in popular culture. Often it is the only novel about cancer that medical students can name.

It is worth bearing in mind that human culture's panoply of literary works is extremely wide-ranging, and that most books which are read by actual readers can be classified as 'popular fiction' rather than 'high art'. While literature by authors such as Tolstoy, Mann, Roth, and de Beauvoir form the basis for our *Writing Cancer* volume, they sell very few copies on the high street or in airport bookshops. Notably, these classical books tend to centre on themes of resilience, gloom, and suffering. With beautiful language, complex psychologies, and elaborate characterisation, their authors seek to evoke difficult emotions and to address profound emotional challenges. Books such as *Love Life*, however, aim for entertainment more than enlightenment. It is not for nothing that readers, in their millions, just find them more *enjoyable*.

Love Life is said to be somewhat autobiographical, although it is a fictionalised version of the experiences of its author, Ray Kluun. Kluun's wife, Judith, died from cancer when he was 36 years old. His novel, which appeared three years after, tells the story of a very similar couple, Dan and Carmen. After Carmen is diagnosed with breast cancer, Dan finds himself incapable of dealing with the emotional turmoil that ensues. Instead he seeks comfort from his drinking buddies and from extramarital sex. He has a passionate affair with Rose, a woman he had spotted on many previous occasions while attending a carnival ("…every year I fall in love with her for three days"; p. 140). When Carmen recovers, Dan admits that he has been sleeping with Rose. The wife forgives him and he, in turn, re-commits himself to her. But ultimately, Carmen becomes ill again and Dan resumes the affair. After Carmen dies by physician-assisted suicide, Dan and Rose's relationship deepens even further (Kim M et al. 2025).

The momentum of *Love Life* is driven by its characters. Dan is a hedonist with self-diagnosed "monophobia", which in this novel is said to be a "morbid fear of a (sexually) monogamous life, leading to a compulsive need for infidelity" (Bamgboje-Ayodele et al. 2021). He works at an ad agency called BBDvW&R/Bernilvy, an alphabet-soup initialism typical of the early years of the new millennium. Sex, drugs, money, and booze feature strongly in his lifestyle. He reacts to news about the results of diagnostic procedures on his wife with phrases based on the lyrics of pop songs. He has at least one sex partner per chapter and at least one trip to Barcelona, New York, or Tel Aviv per month. His daily routine forms the basis of a classic page-turner, especially for readers looking for sex, drugs, and rock 'n' roll—and for easy tears.

Carmen is young and attractive. When she walks into the corridor of the oncology outpatient clinic, "the average age [of those present] plummets by a few decades." It is as though she and Dan are too young, too busy, to be there: "We're clearly new here, we're the waiting-room tourists, and we don't belong here," Dan muses. "But the cancer in Carmen's breast has other ideas" (p. 3).

In one scene, Dan shaves Carmen's head. That way, she still has control over something. But even then, this development is cast in terms of the cosmetic: "She who wants to stay alive must be distinctly ugly. Those are the laws of cancer" (p. 126).

As her illness deteriorates, Carmen writes letters to the couple's two-year-old daughter and openly remarks about the graveyard in which she wishes her corpse to be buried. The thermostat in the living room is set at 24 degrees all day long, and the waterbed is four degrees higher than the recommended temperature. "Any ordinary mattress would be too hard," Dan concludes, as Carmen's body becomes ever more emaciated (p. 281).

Even the doctors are evaluated for their looks and personality. "Dr Scheltema isn't the kind of person who makes you think, 'I bet she's a bit of a laugh'", Dan observes, when he first meets the oncologist. He concludes that she has a "science-geek face" (p. 32). Eventually he goes so far as to seek out a different doctor from another hospital. Dr Jonkman, a man, is also austere, but here Dan finds this comforting. "His words make me start, but I realize he's being so direct deliberately…I like him" (p. 99). When Dan and Carmen explain that their proposed surgeon was actually the same doctor who had misdiagnosed Carmen's condition a year earlier, Dr Jonkman agrees to reschedule the operation so that he can conduct the surgery himself.

While *Love Life* is primarily a romantic drama based on the stereotype of a love triangle, it is not without its subtleties. The English-language title *Love Life* is, itself, a thought-provoking pun—on the one hand, a signifier telling us the story will involve sex; on the other, an exhortation not to waste a single day—a multi-layered title with poignancy as hard-hitting as it is slow-burning. The technicalities of the healthcare system, as well as its pragmatism, are frequently laid bare, providing a backdrop of gentle political commentary that adds authenticity to the reader's experience (Tang et al. 2020). And while the central love triangle consists of Dan, Carmen, and Rose, it is clear that in this novel there is a fourth character at large: cancer, itself, has agency within the story.

The literary quality of *Love Life* may not be what impresses the reader. But the modernity, youth, and jeopardy within its plotline help make the novel compelling. It is hard to blame the author for inauthenticity, given the novel's origins in his own lived experience. And ultimately, the fact that stories such as *Love Life* will find their way into the minds of millions of readers (and movie-goers) means that its gritty account of illness, its focus on couples and the contingency of their commitment, and its consideration of the lives of those who are left behind when someone dies, are certainly worth applauding.

3.30 *Illness as Metaphor*[30]—Susan Sontag

Illness as Metaphor, by the renowned American cultural theorist Susan Sontag (1933–2004), is regarded by many as a classic of its genre. As such, it is all the more interesting to note that it originally appeared not as a single thesis, but as a sequence of three consecutive essays published in the *New York Review of Books*. The integrated volume, which was published in 1978, can be read in many ways: as an intellectual journey through culture in which tuberculosis and cancer play a prominent role; as a manifesto for anti-obscurantism and a philosophical foundation for a thesis on scientific research and the clinical care of people with cancer, in which there is no room for quackery; or, indeed, as a critique of cultural narratives that use cancer as a metaphor for crime, poverty, war, and other social ills, thereby casting misfortune as an unstoppable disease rather than as something subject to human agency (cf., Rieff 2008).

[30] For a recent edition, see: Sontag, S. (2009). *Illness as Metaphor & AIDS and Its Metaphors*. London: Penguin.

Sontag is widely regarded as an influential public intellectual of global significance. Her gravitas was apparent from her writing, but her personal charisma was also obvious in the many recordings of her speeches and readings that can nowadays be found online. When speaking, she sounds like an experienced professor addressing a large lecture hall. Her physical appearance too has an iconic feel. Sontag's bold features were captured in several images by the American photographer Annie Leibovitz, who for many years, including up to Sontag's death, was her closest friend and lover. Strikingly, Sontag's biography contains a photograph taken by Leibovitz showing Sontag's body in a funerary pose shortly after she had died (Leibovitz 2006; Moser 2019).

The cause of Sontag's death was breast cancer, an illness that she kept away from the public eye for a long time. In addition to being a cultural commentary, therefore, *Illness as Metaphor* also serves as Sontag's own version of an illness narrative.

Being ill evokes emotions and cognitions that shape the social appreciation of a disease and its sufferers. The darker the medical explanation for an illness, the darker its social image. According to Sontag, the more unknown the causes and treatment of a disease are said to be, the more prevalent and stigmatising the metaphors associated with it become. Sontag's book examines historical change from the 1800s to the 1900s, focusing on tuberculosis and cancer as the two symbolic illnesses of each century. Sontag shows how both illnesses were widely believed to be associated with the psychological traits of their sufferers. For its part, tuberculosis has long been associated with the suppression of emotions, with dozens of novels describing the introverted typology of the TB sufferer. But, as Sontag argues, these psychosomatic associations became, over time, generalised theories about the nature of the illness itself. TB was not only characterised by emotional suppression, but believed to be *caused* by it.

In reality, the discovery of effective treatments for tuberculosis put paid to claims that the illness was somehow psychogenic. Duly, illness metaphors surrounding TB, and novels that featured them, soon melted away like snow in the sun. It was partly for this reason that, in the twentieth century, a new illness—cancer—became the archetypal object of metaphorical reasoning.

Sontag describes many novels in which psychological cancer metaphors can be found, with cancer linked again to the imperfect regulation of emotion. In this tradition, cancer was associated with "the repression of passion" (p. 23). Sontag mainly cites the work of the Austrian psychoanalyst Wilhelm Reich as having rationalised these notions, presenting the emergence of the metaphor in dozens of novels as a kind of corroboration. If you have cancer, this reasoning proposes, you have your own psychopathology to blame. It is a short leap of logic then to argue that psychotherapy—on its own—can be used as a cancer treatment.

As Sontag suggests, the idea of a specific cancer-prone personality that predisposes human beings to carcinogenesis has been argued by some to be more than a mere metaphor. The claim that psychotherapy can be used on its own to treat such cancer has also been presented by some psychologists, along with datasets that supposedly support the use of talk-based treatments to cure the terminally ill. However, consistent with Sontag's scepticism about these issues, such claims have proved groundless on their face, with the relevant data having been found to be suspect (Pelosi 2019). Today, the claim that psychological therapies can mitigate or reverse the progression of cancer is to be found mainly at the fringes of medical practice, if not beyond the boundary that separates science from pseudoscience (Hughes 2016). Its main downside, apart from the therapies not working, is that the claim shifts the burden of proof from the therapist onto the patient. If an esoteric treatment fails to cure the patient, it can be asserted that it is the patient's fault for having an unsuitable personality. The patient, it can be said, "did not fight hard enough."

On the other hand, personality can go a certain amount of the way, but not by invoking physiological processes that directly cause illness. Instead, a patient's temperament might be pivotal in influencing how they approach the life choices needed to navigate a serious illness. A psychological therapy might then be helpful in improving a patient's focus on their own self-care, or in enhancing their motivation to participate in treatments. After all, a patient whose inclination is to miss their appointments or to forego helpful drugs will likely miss out on whatever advantages medicine has to offer. If some of those advantages include the elimination of cancer, then, in those cases a psychologist who improves their patient's medical motivation can certainly feel validated for having helped them. The patient's personality is the starting point for this chain of events, and, albeit indirectly, influences its outcome.

The idea that it is psychiatric symptomatology that *itself* influences biology in a way that directly steers a patient's cancer—and thus that *psychotherapy* can be deployed to reverse the relevant mechanisms—is, as Sontag suggests, an unhelpful way to think about disease. Not only does it misrepresent the physiology of carcinogenesis, it also discourages and shames cancer patients. Symbolic language assists communication only when it is accurate; when it is inaccurate, understanding is entirely subverted.

If Sontag had written her argument in 2023, she would have found few contemporary novels that portray protagonists as suppressors of passion. Instead, she would have read about themes such as coping, social support, self-management, and cognitive-behavioural therapy. The promotion of mindfulness as a treatment for anxiety and depression in people with cancer might make her smile. Forty years after *Illness as Metaphor* was published, Sontag would have had access to scientific research to incorporate into her argument. At scientific oncology conferences, she could have listened to dozens of lectures on quality of life, a theme that is now at the heart of cancer treatment. She could have read studies on how monitoring quality of life appears to have a positive effect on survival for people with cancer, no doubt because of its positive impact on a patient's motivation to engage constructively with their treatment. Stress reduction too can limit the degree to which stress interferes with immune function, which, in some cases, may complicate some aspects of medical cancer treatments (Antoni and Dhabhar 2019). Furthermore, encouraging physicians to engage emotionally with their patients, to listen to their stories and to empathise with their experiences, enhances the support that they can give to people with cancer.

The trajectory of these new trends of cancer discourse is, in our view, entirely in a positive direction. Sontag was correct that the metaphors used in the nineteenth and twentieth centuries were unhelpful and counterproductive. The shifting of metaphors away from 'cancer-prone personalities' is certainly productive. Instead, as prompted by Sontag, directing attention to ways in which cancer can be thought about truthfully, while still affording patients the dignity they deserve as human beings, is the authentically progressive approach.

We believe that 'blaming the victim' should be replaced by 'patient empowerment.' Furthermore, we believe that patient empowerment is pointless if patients' voices remain unheard. It is for this reason that the written word is so powerful in oncology, as it is in the wider world.

Writing and reading about cancer is therefore not only inherently enlightening. It is integral to the dignity of those who face cancer as well as to their families and loved ones, and absolutely essential to any notion of 'care' (DeShazer 2009).

References

Antoni, M. H., and F. S. Dhabhar. 2019. The impact of psychosocial stress and stress management on immune responses in patients with cancer. *Cancer* 125:1417–1431.

Atkinson, T. M., C. E. Schwartz, L. Goldstein, I. Garcia, D. F. Storfer, Y. Li, J. Zhang, B. H. Bochner, B. D. Rapkin, et al. 2019. Perceptions of response burden associated with completion of patient-reported outcome assessments in oncology. *Value in Health* 22:225–230.

Back, A. L. 2020. Patient-clinician communication issues in palliative care for patients with advanced cancer. *Journal of Clinical Oncology* 38:866–876.

Bamgboje-Ayodele, A., J. V. Levesque, M. Gerges, and A. Girgis. 2021. The male perspective: A mixed methods study of the impact, unmet needs and challenges of caring for women with breast cancer. *Journal of Psychosocial Oncology* 39:235–251.

Bayliss, R. 1998. Pain narratives. In *Narrative medicine*, ed. T. Greenhalgh and B. Hurwitz, 75–82. London: BMJ Press.

Bellon, J. R., H. J. Burstein, E. S. Frank, E. A. Mittendorf, and T. A. King. 2020. Multidisciplinary considerations in the treatment of triple-negative breast cancer. *CA: A Cancer Journal for Clinicians* 70:432–442.

Benson, H., J. A. Dusek, J. B. Sherwood, P. Lam, C. F. Bethea, W. Carpenter, S. Levitsky, P. C. Hill, D. W. Jr. Clem, M. K. Jain, D. Drumel, S. L. Kopecky, P. S. Mueller, D. Marek, S. Rollins, and P. L. Hibberd. 2006. Study of the therapeutic effects of intercessory prayer (STEP) in cardiac bypass patients: A multicenter randomized trial of uncertainty and certainty of receiving intercessory prayer. *American Heart Journal* 151:934–942.

Bergqvist, J., J. H. Nordberg, K. Wode, B. Sunde, P. Fransson, and B. M. Bernhardson. 2025. Living with advanced pancreatic cancer: Patients' experiences of daily life. *Psycho-Oncology* 34:e70260.

Binson, V. A., M. Subramoniam, and L. Mathew. 2021. Discrimination of COPD and lung cancer from controls through breath analysis using a self-developed e-nose. *Journal of Breath Research* 15:046003.

Bishop, M. G. H. 1994. The genius of disease. *Journal of the Royal Society of Medicine* 87:2–4.

Bondevik, H., K. Stene-Johansen, and R. Ahlzén. 2016. Fragments of illness: The death of a beekeeper as a literary case study of cancer. *Medicine Health Care and Philosophy* 19:275–283.

Bremer G. J., and W. Hazeu (red). 1972. Mijn dokter is een goede dokter – poëzie rond het thema ziek-zijn [My doctor is a good doctor – poetry on the theme of being ill]. Lochem: De Tijdstroom.

Brennan, F. 2012. Clock without hands: Carson McCullers and the rhythms of living and dying. *American Journal of Hospice and Palliative Medicine* 30:312–316.

Brennan, M. 2018. Christopher Hitchens' public dying: Toward a secular-humanist ars moriendi? *Omega – Journal of Death and Dying* 77:99–132.

Broadbent, E., J. W. Schoones, J. Tiemensma, and A. A. Kaptein. 2019. A systematic review of patients' drawings of illness: Implications for research using the Common Sense Model. *Health Psychology Review* 13:406–426.

Broyard, B. 2007. *One Drop: My Father's Hidden Life–A Story of Race and Family Secrets*. New York: Little, Brown.

Bukowski C. Carson McCullers. In: The pleasures of the damned. Selected poems, 1951–1993. New York: Harper Collins, 2007, p. 83.

Camidge, R. 2001. Book of the month. *Journal of the Royal Society of Medicine* 94:649–650.

Cassell, E. J. 2004. *The nature of suffering and the goals of medicine*. Oxford: Oxford University Press.

Cuthbert, C. A., J. F. Farragher, B. R. Hemmelgarn, Q. Ding, G. P. McKinnon, and W. Y. Cheung. 2019. Self-management interventions for cancer survivors: A systematic review and evaluation of intervention content and theories. *Psycho-Oncology* 28:2119–2140.

Czerwiec, M. K., and M. N. Huang. 2017. Hospice comics: Representations of patient and family experience of illness and death in graphic novels. *Journal of Medical Humanities* 38:95–113.

Czerwiec, M. K., I. Williams, S. Squier, M. J. Green, K. R. Myers, and S. T. Smith, eds. 2015. *Graphic Medicine Manifesto*. Pennsylvania State University Press: University Park.

Dein, S. 2004. Explanatory models of and attitudes towards cancer in different cultures. *Lancet Oncology* 5:119–124.
DeShazer, M. K. 2009. Cancer narratives and an ethics of commemoration: Susan Sontag, Annie Leibovitz, and David Rieff. *Literature and Medicine* 28:215–236.
Dietl, J. 2004. Thomas Mann's last novella 'The Black Swan': The tragic story of a post-menopausal woman. *European Journal of Obstetrics & Gynecology and Reproductive Biology* 113:255–257.
Ding, P., Q. Zhou, and J. Hu. 2025. Managing psychosocial distress in patients with colorectal cancer. *Medicine* 104:1–4.
Diouri, L., F. Ecarnot, S. Berjot, A. Popiolek, O. Bouche, D. Botsen, et al. 2025. Towards a better understanding of patient expectations: ONCOPREMs-a study – a qualitative study. *Aging Clinical and Experimental Research* 37:256.
Duin, I. A. J., and A. A. Kaptein. 2013. Scared witless about death – Ovarian cancer narratives compared. *Journal of Cancer Education* 28:629–632.
Ehrenreich, B. 2009. *Smile or die: How positive thinking fooled American and the world.* London: Granta.
Eklund, L., M. Engstrōm, A. G. E. M. de Boer, U. Bejerholm, M. Fjell, P. Fessé, et al. 2025. Work-related experiences and needs while undergoing curative cancer therapy: Exploring the target population's perspective during the developmental phase of a work-related intervention. *Supportive Care in Cancer* 33:589.
El-Jawahri, A., D. Forst, A. Fenech, K. O. Brenner, A. L. Jankowski, L. Waldman, I. Sereno, R. Nipp, J. A. Greer, L. Traeger, V. Jackson, and J. Temel. 2020. Relationship between perceptions of treatment goals and psychological distress in patients with advanced cancer. *Journal of the National Comprehensive Cancer Network* 18:849–855.
Elsner, A. M. 2019. Beyond medical paternalism: Undoing the doctor-patient relationship in Simone de Beauvoir's A very easy death. *Literature and Medicine* 37:420–441.
Fang, J., C. Yuan, and B. Suksatit. 2025. Patient-reported emotional responses and coping mechanisms in cancer recurrence: A systematic review of qualitative evidence. *Supportive Care in Cancer* 33:604.
Fauske, L., H. Bondevik, K. Ahlberg, and A. Bjørndal. 2019. Identifying bone sarcoma survivors facing psychosocial challenges. A study of trajectories following treatment. *European Journal of Cancer Care* 28:e13119.
Fitch, M. I. 2020. Exploring experiences of survivors and caregivers regarding lung cancer diagnosis, treatment, and survivorship. *Journal of Patient Experience* 7:193–199.

Florijn, B. W., H. van der Graaf, J. W. Schoones, and A. A. Kaptein. 2019. Narrative medicine: A comparison of terminal cancer patients' stories from a Dutch hospice with those of Anatole Broyard and Christopher Hitchens. *Death Studies* 43:570–581.

Frank, A. W. 1991. *At the will of the body: Reflections on illness*. Boston: Houghton Mifflin Company.

Gates, H. L., Jr. 1996. White like me. *New Yorker*, 66–81, June 17.

Gibson, C., M. O'Connor, R. White, M. Jackson, S. Baxi, and G. K. B. Halkett. 2022. Silenced: Patients' experiences of voicelessness in head and neck cancer. *Patient Education and Counseling* 105:2410–2416.

Gray, J.. 2011. Review: Arguably by Christopher Hitchens. *The New Statesman*, October 6.

Green, M. J., and K. R. Myers. 2010. Graphic medicine: Use of comics in medical education and patient care. *BMJ* 340:574–577.

Greer, J. A., J. M. Jacobs, A. El-Jawahri, R. J. Nipp, E. R. Gallagher, W. F. Pirl, E. R. Park, A. Muzikansky, J. C. Jacobsen, V. A. Jackson, and J. S. Temel. 2018. Role of patient coping strategies in understanding the effects of early palliative care on quality of life and mood. *Journal of Clinical Oncology* 36:53–60.

von Grueningen, V. E., H. Q. Huang, D. Cella, M. A. Zevon, J. A. LaChance, J. L. Walker, R. Salani, S. C. Modesitt, R. T. Morris, W. H. Bradley, W. P. Boente, L. Wenzel, et al. 2018. Quality of life, symptoms and care needs in patients with persistent or recurrent platinum-resistant ovarian cancer: An NRG Oncology/Gynecologic Oncology Group study. *Gynecologic Oncology* 150:119–126.

Hamann, H. A., M. J. Shen, A. J. Thomas, S. J. Craddock Lee, and J. S. Ostroff. 2018a. Development and preliminary psychometric evaluation of a patient-reported outcome measure for lung cancer stigma: The Lung Cancer Stigma Inventory (LCSI). *Stigma Health* 3:195–203.

Hauser, D. J., and N. Schwarz. 2020. The war on prevention II: Battle metaphors undermine cancer treatment and prevention and do not increase vigilance. *Health Communication* 35:1698–1704.

Hilberdink, K. 2007. *Hans Lodeizen – biografie*. Amsterdam: van Oorschot.

Hoerni, B. 2016. Cancer et littérature [Cancer and literature]. *Histoire des Sciences Medicales* 50:199–206.

Hughes, B. M. 2016. *Rethinking psychology: Good science, bad science, pseudoscience*. London: Palgrave.

Hughes, B. M. 2018. *Psychology in crisis*. London: Palgrave.

Hughes, B. 2023. *A conceptual history of psychology: The mind through time.* London: Bloomsbury.
Hunsaker, A. W. 1999. *Reconstructing illness.* West Lafayette: Purdue University Press.
Hutchinson, E. 2001. Book review – *C. Lancet Oncology* 2:321.
Jansen, F., et al. 2019. Stepped care targeting psychological distress in head and neck cancer and lung cancer patients: Which groups specifically benefit? Secondary analyses of a randomized trial. *Supportive Care in Cancer* 27:4543–4553.
Kaptein, A. A. 2022. Novels as data: Health humanities and health psychology. *Journal of Health Psychology* 27:1615–1625.
Kaptein, A. A., and A. C. Lyons. 2010. Cancer ward: Patient perceptions in oncology. *Journal of Health Psychology* 15:848–857.
Kaptein, A. A., and M. S. Y. Thong. 2018. Portraying a grim illness: Lung cancer in novels, poems, films, music, and paintings. *Supportive Cancer Care* 26:3681–3689.
Kaptein, A. A., et al. 2011. Illness perceptions and quality of life in Japanese and Dutch patients with non-small cell lung cancer. *Lung Cancer* 72:384–390.
Kaptein, A. A., et al. 2013. Illness perceptions and quality of life in Japanese and Dutch women with breast cancer. *Journal of Psychosocial Oncology* 31:83–102.
Kaptein, A. A., B. M. Hughes, M. Murray, and J. M. Smyth. 2018. Start making sense. Art informing health psychology. *Health Psychology Open* 10:1–13.
Kaptein, A. A., W. E. Hanser, J. W. Schoones, P. Boot, J. W. Pennebaker, and B. M. Hughes. 2025. Cancer in poetry – poetry in cancer: A linguistic analysis of poems by poets on their own cancer and on the cancer of their loved ones. *Psycho-Oncology* 34 (10): e70297.
Kedia, S. K., et al. 2019. Psychosocial interventions for informal caregivers of lung cancer patients: A systematic review. *Psycho-oncology* 29:251–262.
Kharade, P., et al. 2018. Appraisal of function after rehabilitation with tongue prosthesis. *Journal of Craniofacial Surgery* 29:e41–e44.
Kim, M., K. Tan, and L. A. Coombs. 2025. Effects of web-based interventions on cancer caregivers' burden and quality of life: A systematic review and et-analysis. *Palliative and Supportive Care* 23:e134.
Kleijn, G., B. I. Lissenberg-Witte, E. Bohlmeijer, V. Willemsen, A. Becker-Commissaris, C. M. Eeltink, A. M. E. Bruynzeel, M. J. van der Vorst, P. Cuijpers, and I. M. Verdonck-de Leeuw. 2021. A randomized controlled trial on the efficacy of life review therapy targeting incurably ill cancer patients: Do their informal caregivers benefit? *Supportive Care in Cancer* 29:1257–1264.

Körner, A., N. Roberts, R. J. Steele, D. C. Brosseau, and Z. Rosberger. 2019. A randomized controlled trial assessing the efficacy of a self-administered psycho-educational intervention for patients with cancer. *Patient Education and Counseling* 102:735–741.

Lahtinen, A. M., and M. Torppa. 2007. 'Medicalisation of falling in love': Medical students' responses to Thomas Mann's The Black Swan. *Medical Humanities* 33:44–48.

Lambert, S. D., L. O. Brahim, M. Morrison, A. Girgis, M. Yaffe, E. Belzile, K. Clayberg, J. Robinson, S. Thorne, J. L. Bottorff, W. Duggleby, H. Campbell-Enns, K. Youngmee, and C. G. Loiselle. 2019. Priorities for caregiver research in cancer care: An international Delphi survey of caregivers, clinicians, managers, and researchers. *Supportive Care in Cancer* 27:805–817.

Lawson, D. 2001. Introduction. In *Snake oil and other preoccupations*, ed. J. Diamond. London: Vintage.

Lefkovits, Y. R., N. Heriot, A. Sporik, S. Perera, M. Friedlander, C. Dixon, et al. 2024. Incorporating patient-reported outcome measures (PROMs) into a clinical quality registry (CQR) for ovarian cancer: Considerations and challenges. *BMC Health Services Research* 24:778.

Leibovitz, A. 2006. *A photographers' life 1990–2005*. New York: Random House.

Levinsen, A. K. G, S. O. Dalton, E. Jakobsen, I. Gögenur, M. Borre, and R. Zachariae, et al. In Press. Prevalence of and factors associated with clinically important levels of fatigue, pain, and insomnia in survivors of cancer: A population-based cross-sectional study. *Journal of Cancer Survivorship*.

Linklater, A.. 2012. Mortality by Christopher Hitchens: Review. *The Observer*, August 26.

Liu, F., H. Shan, W. Bing, L. Sun, and L. Wei. 2025. Relationship between symptom burden and benefit finding in patients with gastrointestinal cancers undergoing chemotherapy: The chain-mediating role of comprehensive needs and communication pattern. *Supportive Care in Cancer* 33:816.

Ljunggren, B. 1993. Herbert Olivecrona: Founder of Swedish neurosurgery. *Journal of Neurosurgery* 78:142–149.

Lo-Fo-Wong, D., A. Beijaerts, H. C. J. M. de Haes, and M. A. G. Sprangers. 2014. Cancer in full-colour: Use of a graphic novel to identify distress in women with breast cancer. *Journal of Health Psychology* 19:1554–1563.

Lorde, A. 1983. There is no hierarchy of oppressions. *Interracial Books for Children Bulletin* 14 (3–4): 9.

Łuczyk, R. J., K. Sikora, A. Bodio, M. Łuczyk, M. Baryła-Matejczuk, A. Wawryniuk, et al. 2024. Role of emotional control on anxiety and stress among cancer patients. *Cancer Medicine* 13:e70162.

Mäkitie, A. A., R. O. Alabi, L. Pulkki-Råback, A. Almangush, J. J. Beitler, N. F. Saba, et al. 2024. Psychological factors related to treatment outcomes in head and neck cancer. *Advances in Therapy* 41:3489–3519.

McCurry, J. 2015. Hiroshima survivors remember. *Lancet* 386:417–418.

McMullin, J. 2016. Cancer and the Comics: Graphic narratives and biolegitimate lives. *Medical Anthropology Quarterly* 30:149–167.

McNeil, C. M. 2018. Grace and forgiveness. *Journal of Clinical Oncology* 36:1045–1046.

Merz, E. L., R. S. Fox, and V. L. Malcarne. 2014. Expressive writing interventions in cancer patients: A systematic review. *Health Psychology Review* 8:339–361.

Miller, M., M. Meyers, K. Krainak, and S. P. Lewis. 2025. Interventions to support spirituality among adults with cancer: A scoping review. *Supportive Care in Cancer* 33:742.

Miranda, K. W., B. L. Musher, and H. J. Badr. 2025. Unmet supportive care needs in patients with advanced cancer and its impact on distress. *BMC Palliative Care* 24:110.

Moreno-Alonso, D., B. G. García, C. Madrid-Alejos, G. Morón-Cazalilla, S. Llorens-Torromé, I. Crespo, et al. 2025. Bridging the gap: An updated systematic integrative review of palliative care integration in hematological malignancies. *Seminars in Oncology Nursing* xxx:151962.

Moser, B. 2019. *Sontag – her life*. New York: Harper Collins.

Naef, A. P., and E. William. 1998. Adams: Thomas Mann and The Magic Mountain. *Annals of Thoracic Surgery* 65:285–287.

Naono, A. 2019. The origins of 'Hibakusha' as a scientific and political classification of the survivor. *Japanese Studies* 39:333–352.

Niscola, P., D. Piccioni, and M. Giovannini. 2025. Palliative care interventions and their early integration in the management of older adults with acute myeloid leukaemia: A narrative review. *Annals of Palliative Medicine* 14:393–411.

Nisiraiou, A., A. Bozas, D. Kyrou, K. Stavrogianni, M. M. Vasilopoulou, G. M. Kalomoiris, et al. 2025. Post-traumatic growth in adult cancer survivors: A scoping review of psychological factors, predictors, and interventions. *International Journal of Psychiatry* 60:e70097.

Nogueria, C. M., B. S. Reis, A. de F. R. Meneses, B. H. Mellado, and Reis FJC. 2025. Unveiling delays: Understanding the diagnostic pathways of women with advanced cervical cancer. *Supportive Care in Cancer* 33:826.

Oates J. C. 2017. The poet of freakiness. *New York Review of Books*, September 28, 78–80.

Olson, L. 2011. Anger among allies: Audre Lorde's 1981 keynote admonishing the National Women's Studies Association. *Quarterly Journal of Speech* 97 (3): 283–308.

Orr, L. D., J. Vanderpoel, P. Vadagam, M. I. Patel, U. B. Roy, B. Ledezma, et al. 2025. Patient, care partner, and provider voice in treatment decision-making for non-small cell lung cancer. *Patient Education and Counseling* 136:108776.

Paulson, A. E., A. Stein, J. K. Kendal, N. M. Bernthal, and L. E. Wessel. 2024. Most patients with bone sarcomas seek emotional support and information about other patients' experiences: A thematic analysis. *Clinical Orthopedic Related Research* 482:161–171.

Pelosi, A. J. 2019. Personality and fatal diseases: Revisiting a scientific scandal. *Journal of Health Psychology* 24:421–439.

Pereira, N. R. P., S. J. Janssen, N. Stoop, S. Hartvelt, Y. Chen, T. F. DeLaney, F. J. Hornicek, and J. H. Schwab. 2019. Physical function and quality of life after resection of mobile spine chondrosarcoma. *Global Spine Journal* 9:743–753.

Philipp, R., A. Mehnert, C. Lo, V. Mueler, M. Reck, and S. Vehling. 2019. Characterizing death acceptance among patients with cancer. *Psycho-Oncology* 28:854–862.

Porter, L. S., G. Samsa, J. L. Steel, L. C. Hanson, T. W. LeBlanc, J. Bull, S. Fischer, and F. J. Keefe. 2019. Caregiver-guided pain coping skills training for patients with advanced cancer: Background, design, and challenges for the CaringPals study. *Clinical Trials* 16:262–272.

Post, K. E., S. Aribindi, L. Traeger, D. Hall, J. Jacobs, J. S. Temel, et al. 2025. Not out of the woods: Perspectives from patients with triple-negative breast cancer. *Supportive Care in Cancer* 33:18.

Richardson, A. E., E. Broadbent, and R. P. Morton. 2019. A systematic review of psychological interventions for patients with head and neck cancer. *Supportive Care in Cancer* 27:2007–2021.

Rieff, D. 2008. *Swimming in a sea of death: A son's memoir*. New York: Simon & Schuster.

Riskin, J. 2016. *The restless clock: A history of the centuries-long argument over what makes living things tick*. Chicago: University of Chicago Press.

Romagna, A., C. Schwartz, B. Huffman, W. Hitzl, R. A. Kristof, H. Clusmann, and C. Blume. 2025. Analysis of quality of life and outcomes of vestibular schwannoma patients after resection and radiosurgery in an interdisciplinary treatment concept. *Nature Scientific Reports* 15:15941.

Ruben, M. A., D. Blanch-Hartigan, and J. C. Shipherd. 2018. To know another's pain: A meta-analysis of caregivers' and healthcare providers' pain assessment accuracy. *Annals of Behavioral Medicine* 52:662–685.

Sabin, R. 1996. *Comics, Comix & Graphic Novels*. New York: Phaidon Press.
Samuel J. N., Booth, C. M., Eisenhauer, E., Brundage, M., Berry, S. R., and Gyawali, B. 2022. Association of quality-of-life outcomes in cancer drug trials with survival outcomes and drug class. *JAMA Oncolology* 1:879–886.
Sánchez-Gómez, C., E. J. Fernández-Rodriguez, S. Jiménez-Sánchez, E. Fonseca-Sánchez, J. Perez, V. Navarro-López, et al. 2025. Effect of cognitive training on cancer-related cognitive impairment in patients with breast cancer: A systematic review and meta-analysis. *Psycho-Oncology* 34:e70251.
Schmidt, N. 2018. Intertextuality and the transnational in Verena Stefan's Fremdschläfer (2007): Writing breast cancer from beyond the border. In *The wounded self, writing illness in twenty-first-century German literature*, ed. N. Schmidt, 92–113. Rochester NY: Camden House.
Sisi, Y., C. Yao, K. Yajuan, S. Suting, J. Du, H. Qu, et al. 2025. Pulmonary rehabilitation for patients receiving lung cancer radiotherapy: A scoping review. *BMJ Open* 15:e091749.
Slawson, D. C., and A. F. Shaughnessy. 1997. Obtaining useful information from expert based sources. *BMJ* 314:947–953.
Sontag, S. 1978. *Illness as metaphor*. New York: Farrar, Straus Giroux.
Sowell, F. G., T. de Milliano, K. J. S. Brady, G. Foglia, M. Sasane, S. Bensfia, et al. 2025. A conceptual model for advanced/metastatic gastric or gastroesophageal junction cancer: A review of qualitative studies and results from patient interviews. *BMC Cancer* 25:88.
Staples, B. 2003. Editorial observer; back when skin color was destiny–unless you passed for white. *New York Times*, September 7.
Swain, K. 2017. Podcast: The Chemo files: One year on. *Lancet Oncology* 18:179.
Tang, M., X. Liu, Q. Wu, and Y. Shi. 2020. The effects of cognitive-behavioral stress management for breast cancer patients. *Cancer Nursing* 43:222–237.
Temel, J., J. A. Greer, A. Muzikansky, E. R. Gallagher, S. Admane, V. A. Jackson, C. M. Dahlin, C. D. Blindermann, J. Jacobsen, W. F. Pirl, J. A. Billings, and T. J. Lynch. 2010. Early palliative care for patients with metastatic non-small-cell lung cancer. *New England Journal of Medicine* 363:733–742.
Terayama, T., J. Shigemura, Y. Kobayashi, M. Kurosawa, M. Nagamine, H. Toda, et al. 2021. Mental health consequences for survivors of the 2011 Fukushima nuclear disaster: A systematic review. Part 2: Emotional and behavioral consequences. *CNS Spectrums* 26:30–42.
Timmermann, C. 2014. *A history of lung cancer. The recalcitrant disease*. New York: Palgrave.

Tsiakiri, A., A. Despoti, P. Koutsimani, K. Megari, S. Plakias, and A. Tsapanou. 2025. Mapping cognitive oncology: A decade of trends and research fronts. *Medical Sciences* 13:19.

Tundealao, S., P. Okunlola, O. Alabaku, O. Noah, O. Alufa, and T. Titiloye. 2025. Head and neck related quality of life following glossectomy among tongue cancer patients: A systematic review and meta-analysis. *Oral and Maxillofacial Surgery* 29:164.

Turkman, Y. E., H. P. Kennedy, L. N. Harris, and M. T. Knobf. 2016. 'An addendum to breast cancer': The triple negative experience. *Supportive Care in Cancer* 24:3715–3721.

Twiddy, I. 2015. *Cancer poetry*. Basingstoke: Palgrave Macmillan.

Updike, J. 1982. From the journal of a leper. *American Journal of Dermatopathology* 4:137–142.

Verghese, A. 2020. Writing medicine. *JAMA* 323:1649–1650.

Vestdijk, S. 1964. *De zieke mens in de romanliteratuur [The ill person in literature]*. Delft: Koninklijke Nederlandse Gist – en Spiritusfabriek.

von Engelhardt, D. 2021a. Cancer in literature: Between phenomenology and symbolism. In *Ethical challenges in cancer diagnosis and therapy*, ed. A. W. Bauer et al., 275–290. Zurich: Springer Nature Switzerland.

Watson, J., C. S. Peng, M. Desir, M. N. Mate-Cole, and H. Amonoo. 2025. Expressive writing interventions in patients with cancer: A scoping literature review. *Palliative and Supportive Care* 23 (e132): 1–20.

Whitt, J. 1999. The "we of me": Carson McCullers as lesbian novelist. *Journal of Homosexuality* 37:127–139.

Williams, I. C. M. 2012. Graphic medicine: Comics as medical narrative. *Medical Humanities* 38:21–27.

Wu, T. J., C. S. Sheih, S. T. Jou, C. Y. Lee, T. Y. Yu, C. Y. Liu, and C. W. Chen. 2025. Effects of bibliotherapy on emotional distress, coping strategies, and resilience in adolescents with cancer: A pilot randomized controlled trial. *European Journal of Oncology Nursing* 76:102900.

Xiang, J., L. Dai, L. Tan, D. Lv, Y. Chen, L. Tang, et al. 2025. Psychosocial experiences of prostate cancer survivors after treatment: A systematic review of qualitative studies. *Frontiers in Public Health* 13:1625611.

Zulman, D. M., M. C. Haverfield, J. G. Shaw, C. G. Brown-Johnson, R. Schwartz, A. A. Tierney, D. L. Zionts, N. Safaeinili, M. Fischer, Israni S. Thadaney, S. M. Asch, and A. Verghese. 2020. Practices to foster physician presence and connection with patients in the clinical encounter. *JAMA* 323:70–81.

4

Living Cancer

It is relatively easy to find tens, if not hundreds, of novels, pieces of reportage, and other forms of creative writing that address issues arising from cancer. They can be encountered almost anywhere—in 'high art' writing, popular fiction, historical literature, or graphic novels. The word *cancer* has an immediate resonance for most listeners. The topic has inspired literally millions of written words. Indeed, the selection presented in this book represents but a fraction of what is available. Many additional works could have been incorporated (and may perhaps warrant a follow-up volume), including the Irish-born poet Lucy Grealy's *Autobiography of a Face* (1994), which recalled her experience in childhood of Ewing's sarcoma that left her jaw permanently disfigured. Jane Kenyon's collection, *Otherwise: New and Selected Poems* (1996), which she was still compiling when she died of cancer, could also have been considered, as well as the book of poetry written by her husband Donald Hall, *Without* (1999), two volumes that together poignantly describe the emotional, practical, and interpersonal challenges facing couples who are living shared lives while one of them is dying. Other works worthy of honourable mentions include Reynolds Price's memoir *A Whole New Life: An Illness and a Healing* (1994), which chronicled the poet's journey

A. A. Kaptein, B. M. Hughes, *Writing Cancer*,
https://doi.org/10.1007/978-981-95-6501-6_4

from cancer diagnosis to spinal surgery and his eventual paralysis as a result, as well as the actor Evan Handler's books *Time On Fire: My Comedy of Terrors* (1996) and *It's Only Temporary…The Good News and the Bad News of Being Alive* (2008), which together describe the personal journey of a young man in his twenties through acute myeloid leukaemia. Recently, a publication offered an empirical study on poems about cancer based on a database of some 130 poems on cancer by poets who had cancer and by poets describing the cancer of their loved ones, analysed with the Linguistic Inquiry and Word Count methodology (Kaptein et al. 2025).

One puzzle is why cancer, specifically, occupies this role of artistic muse. The prevalence of cancer as an illness is undoubtedly a factor. But ultimately, what drives creative literature is not disease prevalence in statistical terms, but illness perceptions in psychological terms. It is the social appreciation of cancer that determines how many novels get written. The psychological impacts of various diseases differ, a diversity that should fascinate the general public as well as medical psychologists. And it is these impacts that determine dramatic value. For example, cancer is frequently disfiguring, sudden, mysterious, and unavoidable, making it an archetypal adversary for fiction. Cardiovascular disease, on the other hand, is often none of those things. Cardiology is also way ahead of oncology in providing effective therapeutic measures. And as Sontag observed, once effective treatments are established for an illness, it because less interesting. Associated 'myths' dissipate.

Illness narratives and novels often centre upon suffering, which may make cancer a more usable disease for fiction. But rheumatoid arthritis also creates a lot of painful suffering, as do many respiratory illnesses. Chronic back pain is also a prominent medical cause of human misery. But the biological processes underlying such conditions are often hidden from view—many people with chronic pain look identical to people without it—potentially leading these ailments to be perceived as less dramatic than cancer. What Susan Sontag points out about disease may also play a role: cancer is seen as a scientific challenge, and the search for a cure is an important human quest. If an effective generic cancer treatment can be found, the illness may lose its dramatic gravitas, as tuberculosis did in the past (Hughes 2023; Sontag 1978).

The literary works discussed in this volume represent a wide range of subjects. But what is clear is that when authors write about cancer, they are focusing on more than just mortality. Mortality is certainly a salient subject of interest, but the human experience of cancer ranges widely. In that sense, the fact that heart disease kills more people each year is hardly relevant. There is more to disease than death.

With that in mind, the creative arts, and literature in particular, have the potential to offer important insights into cancer that lie far beyond what can be derived from biomedicine. It is true that works of literature are akin to anecdotal evidence in scientific terms: they provide testimonies from narrators (many of them purely fictional) rather than data that can be measured and analysed. However, literature will not rise to prominence if it fails to resonate with readers. As such, what we find in works of literature constitutes a type of *cultural* data. It helps us understand how the experience of cancer is processed by human minds. It offers a starting point for considerations of dimensions of experience that might otherwise go unnoticed. For example, an interesting assignment for medical students, especially trainee medical oncologists, would be to assess the various works discussed in this book in terms of whether their authors have pursued a primarily biomedical or biopsychosocial emphasis. It is helpful to know which of these readers are actually attracted to.

Ultimately, given the mass appeal of talented writing, such literature also helps to communicate these ideas to the wider world. In this way, those who engage in the activity of 'writing cancer' can contribute to our collective understanding in important ways that would be difficult for psychologists to do with their customary research data.

Some might hesitate to promote the value of cancer literature in this way. After all, our opinions here are framed by a relatively narrow range of cultural outputs, with the majority of works reflecting European and North American cultural norms. Literary works written from other cultural perspectives lie outside our review. And of course, our selection is far from systematic. Our personal preferences and dislikes played a role in our choices. But once again, the idea here is to provide a meaningful perspective on the issues as we find them, rather than a systematically analysed dataset.

Another limitation is that the novels have not been analysed with knowledge and theories from the literary sciences. We are not, and do not purport to be, literary scholars. Moreover, we are sure that literary expertise would only enhance the potential of this type of work. We would be delighted if literary scholars could apply their skills and insights to further mine this body of written literature. In the meantime, we humbly offer our take on things, hoping that our understanding and experience of medical psychology will ensure that something useful is contributed. It is our hope that the field referred to as 'medical humanities' continues not only to expand, but also to deepen.

Within the mainstream of psychological science, we also hope that future research can examine ways to develop and refine methods for analysing novels (as well as other art genres). Whether this could be assisted by new forms of AI is for others to determine. Currently, it is difficult to systematically examine the existing databases to locate creative writing that deals with cancer in general, let alone different discrete categories of cancer.

While bibliotherapy and related approaches can be of benefit in clinical practice, we feel that the consideration of literary works offers huge potential in medical education. Nothing produces authentic perspective-taking as much as immersing yourself in an author's universe. There is something inherent in human psychology that enables readers to become gripped by a dramatic narrative, something that can never be tapped by pedagogical prose. Reading what someone has written about cancer, from direct or vicarious personal experience, creates a type of connection that all clinicians struggle to form with their patients. In our view, every medical student should read such works as part of their training.

In one of our *Literature & Medicine* honours classes, medical students were guided to study cancer from a biopsychosocial perspective. Their assignment consisted of three parts. They were to study the formal biomedical background of a disease (specifically, gastric carcinoma). They were then to study a novel in which gastric carcinoma plays a prominent role. Finally they were instructed to listen to a patient with gastric carcinoma talking about their experience (and to do so, if possible, in the patient's own home). The three tasks were then to be integrated into a single manuscript describing what the student had learned. The task yielded some truly beautiful student work, with a profundity that far exceeded the sum of its parts. This three-pillared approach can of course also be applied to a clinician's own practice, without their having to write a manuscript about it (and patients too could perhaps be invited to read the same works as their clinician).

Overall, we feel that *reading* cancer should form part of every physician's ongoing professional development. In our view, the communion of human thought that is achieved by *Writing Cancer* is what makes it a perennial, and essential, cultural activity.

References

Hughes, B. 2023. *A conceptual history of psychology: The mind through time.* London: Bloomsbury.

Kaptein, A. A., W. E. Hanser, J. W. Schoones, P. Boot, J. W. Pennebaker, and B. M. Hughes. 2025. Cancer in poetry – poetry in cancer: A linguistic analysis of poems by poets on their own cancer and on the cancer of their loved ones. *Psycho-Oncology* 34 (10): e70297.

Sontag, S. 1978. *Illness as metaphor*. New York: Farrar, Straus Giroux.

References

Antoni, M. H., and F. S. Dhabhar. 2019. The impact of psychosocial stress and stress management on immune responses in patients with cancer. *Cancer* 125:1417–1431.

Aronson, J. K. 2000. Autopathography: The patient's tale. *BMJ* 321:1599–1602.

Atkinson, T. M., C. E. Schwartz, L. Goldstein, I. Garcia, D. F. Storfer, Y. Li, J. Zhang, B. H. Bochner, B. D. Rapkin, et al. 2019. Perceptions of response burden associated with completion of patient-reported outcome assessments in oncology. *Value in Health* 22:225–230.

Atkinson, T. M., A. C. Dueck, D. V. Satele, G. Thanarajasingam, J. M. Lafky, J. A. Sloan, and E. Basch. 2020. Clinician vs patient reporting of baseline and postbaseline symptoms for adverse event assessment in cancer clinical trials. *JAMA Oncology* 6:437–439.

Back, A. L. 2020. Patient-clinician communication issues in palliative care for patients with advanced cancer. *Journal of Clinical Oncology* 38:866–876.

Bamgboje-Ayodele, A., J. V. Levesque, M. Gerges, and A. Girgis. 2021. The male perspective: A mixed methods study of the impact, unmet needs and challenges of caring for women with breast cancer. *Journal of Psychosocial Oncology* 39:235–251.

Basch, E., L. Wilfong, and D. Schrag. 2020. Adding patient-reported outcomes to medicare's oncology value-based payment model. *JAMA* 323:213–214.

A. A. Kaptein, B. M. Hughes, *Writing Cancer*,
https://doi.org/10.1007/978-981-95-6501-6

Bates, V., A. Bleakley, and S. Goodman, eds. 2014. *Medicine, health and the arts – approaches to the medical humanities*. London: Routledge.

Bauereiss, N., S. Obermaier, S. E. Özünal, and H. Baumeister. 2018. Effects of existential interventions on spiritual, psychological, and physical well-being in adult patients with cancer: Systematic review and meta-analysis of randomized controlled trials. *Psycho-Oncology* 27:2531–2545.

Bayliss, R. 1998. Pain narratives. In *Narrative medicine*, ed. T. Greenhalgh and B. Hurwitz, 75–82. London: BMJ Press.

Bellon, J. R., H. J. Burstein, E. S. Frank, E. A. Mittendorf, and T. A. King. 2020. Multidisciplinary considerations in the treatment of triple-negative breast cancer. *CA: A Cancer Journal for Clinicians* 70:432–442.

Benson, H., J. A. Dusek, J. B. Sherwood, P. Lam, C. F. Bethea, W. Carpenter, S. Levitsky, P. C. Hill, D. W. Jr. Clem, M. K. Jain, D. Drumel, S. L. Kopecky, P. S. Mueller, D. Marek, S. Rollins, and P. L. Hibberd. 2006. Study of the therapeutic effects of intercessory prayer (STEP) in cardiac bypass patients: A multicenter randomized trial of uncertainty and certainty of receiving intercessory prayer. *American Heart Journal* 151:934–942.

Bergqvist, J., J. H. Nordberg, K. Wode, B. Sunde, P. Fransson, and B. M. Bernhardson. 2025. Living with advanced pancreatic cancer: Patients' experiences of daily life. *Psycho-Oncology* 34:e70260.

Bernhardsson, K. 2010. *Litterära besvär [Suffering in literature]*. Stockholm: Ellerströms.

Binson, V. A., M. Subramoniam, and L. Mathew. 2021. Discrimination of COPD and lung cancer from controls through breath analysis using a self-developed e-nose. *Journal of Breath Research* 15:046003.

Bishop, M. G. H. 1994. The genius of disease. *Journal of the Royal Society of Medicine* 87:2–4.

Bleakley, A. 2015. *Medical humanities and medical education*. London: Routledge.

Bleakley, A., and S. Neilson. 2022. *Poetry in the clinic – towards a lyrical medicine*. London: Routledge.

Boland, L., K. Bennett, and D. Connolly. 2018. Self-management interventions for cancer survivors: A systematic review. *Supportive Care in Cancer* 26:1585–1595.

Bondevik, H., K. Stene-Johansen, and R. Ahlzén. 2016. Fragments of illness: The death of a beekeeper as a literary case study of cancer. *Medicine Health Care and Philosophy* 19:275–283.

Bone, J. K., D. Fancourt, J. K. Sonke, and F. Bu. 2024. Participatory and receptive arts engagement in older adults: Associations with cognition over a seven-year period. *Creativity Research Journal* 36:436–450.

Boyer, A. 2019. *The undying*. New York: Farrar, Straus and Giroux.

Bradt, J., C. Dileo, K. Myers-Coffman, and J. Biondo. 2021. Music interventions for improving psychological and physical outcomes in people with cancer (review). *Cochrane Database of Systematic Reviews* 10 (10): CD006911.

Bremer G. J., and W. Hazeu (red). 1972. Mijn dokter is een goede dokter – poëzie rond het thema ziek-zijn [My doctor is a good doctor – poetry on the theme of being ill]. Lochem: De Tijdstroom.

Brennan, F. 2012. Clock without hands: Carson McCullers and the rhythms of living and dying. *American Journal of Hospice and Palliative Medicine* 30:312–316.

Brennan, M. 2018. Christopher Hitchens' public dying: Toward a secular-humanist ars moriendi? *Omega – Journal of Death and Dying* 77:99–132.

Broadbent, E., J. W. Schoones, J. Tiemensma, and A. A. Kaptein. 2019. A systematic review of patients' drawings of illness: Implications for research using the Common Sense Model. *Health Psychology Review* 13:406–426.

Brody, H. 1973. The systems view of man: Implications for medicine, science, and ethics. *Perspectives in Biology and Medicine* 17:71–92.

Broyard, A. 1992. *Intoxicated by my illness*. New York: Clarkson Potter.

Broyard, B. 2007. *One Drop: My Father's Hidden Life–A Story of Race and Family Secrets*. New York: Little, Brown.

Bukowski C. Carson McCullers. In: The pleasures of the damned. Selected poems, 1951–1993. New York: Harper Collins, 2007, p. 83.

Butler, D. J. 2009. Teaching about the traumatic impact of vehicular crashes: Rock 'n roll never forgets. *Family Medicine* 41:549–551.

Calne, R. 1996. *Art, surgery and transplantation*. London: Williams & Wilkins.

Camidge, R. 2001. Book of the month. *Journal of the Royal Society of Medicine* 94:649–650.

Caminiti, C., M. A. Annunziata, C. Verusio, C. Pinto, M. Airoldi, et al. 2021. Effectiveness of a psychosocial care quality improvement strategy to address quality of life in patients with cancer. *JAMA Network Open* 4:1–14.

Cassell, E. J. 2004. *The nature of suffering and the goals of medicine*. Oxford: Oxford University Press.

Charon, R. 2010. Calculating the contributions of Humanities to medical practice – motives, methods, and metrics. *Academic Medicine* 85:935–937.

Clift, S., and K. Grebosz-Haring. 2025. The need for a critical perspective on arts and health research and reviews. Comment on "Can arts-based interventions improve health? A conceptual and methodological critique" by Martin Skov and Marcos Nadal. *Physics of Life Reviews* 54:116–119.

Crawford, P., B. Brown, C. Baker, V. Tischler, and B. Abrams, eds. 2015. *Health humanities*. London: Palgrave.

Cuthbert, C. A., J. F. Farragher, B. R. Hemmelgarn, Q. Ding, G. P. McKinnon, and W. Y. Cheung. 2019. Self-management interventions for cancer survivors: A systematic review and evaluation of intervention content and theories. *Psycho-Oncology* 28:2119–2140.

Czerwiec, M. K., and M. N. Huang. 2017. Hospice comics: Representations of patient and family experience of illness and death in graphic novels. *Journal of Medical Humanities* 38:95–113.

Czerwiec, M. K., I. Williams, S. Squier, M. J. Green, K. R. Myers, and S. T. Smith, eds. 2015. *Graphic Medicine Manifesto*. Pennsylvania State University Press: University Park.

Dalrymple, T., ed. 2021. *The best medicine – Stories of healing*. New York: A.A. Knopf.

Darbyshire, D., and P. Baker. 2012. A systematic review and thematic analysis of cinema in medical education. *Medical Humanities* 38:28–33.

De Beauvoir, S. 1965. *A very easy death*. New York: Pantheon Books.

Dein, S. 2004. Explanatory models of and attitudes towards cancer in different cultures. *Lancet Oncology* 5:119–124.

DeShazer, M. K. 2009. Cancer narratives and an ethics of commemoration: Susan Sontag, Annie Leibovitz, and David Rieff. *Literature and Medicine* 28:215–236.

Detmar, S. B., M. J. Muller, J. H. Schornagel, L. D. V. Wever, and N. K. Aaronson. 2002. Health-related quality-of-life assessments and patient-physician communication. *JAMA* 288:3027–3034.

Diamond, J. 1998. *C: Because cowards get cancer too ….* London: Vermillion.

Dietl, J. 2004. Thomas Mann's last novella 'The Black Swan': The tragic story of a post-menopausal woman. *European Journal of Obstetrics & Gynecology and Reproductive Biology* 113:255–257.

Ding, P., Q. Zhou, and J. Hu. 2025. Managing psychosocial distress in patients with colorectal cancer. *Medicine* 104:1–4.

Diouri, L., F. Ecarnot, S. Berjot, A. Popiolek, O. Bouche, D. Botsen, et al. 2025. Towards a better understanding of patient expectations: ONCOPREMs-a study – a qualitative study. *Aging Clinical and Experimental Research* 37:256.

Diski, J. 2016. *In gratitude*. London: Bloomsbury.

Duin, I. A. J., and A. A. Kaptein. 2013. Scared witless about death – Ovarian cancer narratives compared. *Journal of Cancer Education* 28:629–632.

Edson, M. 1993. *Wit*. New York: Farrar, Straus and Giroux.

Ehrenreich, B. 2009. *Smile or die: How positive thinking fooled American and the world*. London: Granta.

Eklund, L., M. Engström, A. G. E. M. de Boer, U. Bejerholm, M. Fjell, P. Fessé, et al. 2025. Work-related experiences and needs while undergoing curative cancer therapy: Exploring the target population's perspective during the developmental phase of a work-related intervention. *Supportive Care in Cancer* 33:589.

El-Jawahri, A., D. Forst, A. Fenech, K. O. Brenner, A. L. Jankowski, L. Waldman, I. Sereno, R. Nipp, J. A. Greer, L. Traeger, V. Jackson, and J. Temel. 2020. Relationship between perceptions of treatment goals and psychological distress in patients with advanced cancer. *Journal of the National Comprehensive Cancer Network* 18:849–855.

Elkington, J. R. 1966. Medicine and the quality of life. *Annals of Internal Medicine* 64:711–714.

Elsner, A. M. 2019. Beyond medical paternalism: Undoing the doctor-patient relationship in Simone de Beauvoir's A very easy death. *Literature and Medicine* 37:420–441.

Engel, G. L. 1977. The need for a new medical model: A challenge for biomedicine. *Science* 196:129–136.

von Engelhardt, D. 2021a. Cancer in literature: Between phenomenology and symbolism. In *Ethical challenges in cancer diagnosis and therapy*, ed. A. W. Bauer et al., 275–290. Zurich: Springer Nature Switzerland.

von Engelhardt, D. 2021b. *Medizin der Literatur der Neuzeit [Literature and Medicine in modern time]. Band 1 to 5*. Heidelberg: Mattes Verlag.

Fancourt, D. 2026. *Art cure: The science of how the arts transform our health*. Cornerstone Press.

Fang, J., C. Yuan, and B. Suksatit. 2025. Patient-reported emotional responses and coping mechanisms in cancer recurrence: A systematic review of qualitative evidence. *Supportive Care in Cancer* 33:604.

Fares, C. M., T. J. Williamson, M. K. Theisen, A. Cummings, K. Bornazyan, M. L. Carroll, A. L. Stanton, and E. B. Garon. 2018. Low concordance of patient-reported outcomes with clinical and clinical trial documentation. *Journal of Clinical Oncology* 2:1–12.

Fauske, L., H. Bondevik, K. Ahlberg, and A. Bjørndal. 2019. Identifying bone sarcoma survivors facing psychosocial challenges. A study of trajectories following treatment. *European Journal of Cancer Care* 28:e13119.

Fies, B. 2006. *Mom's Cancer*. New York: Abrams.

Fitch, M. I. 2020. Exploring experiences of survivors and caregivers regarding lung cancer diagnosis, treatment, and survivorship. *Journal of Patient Experience* 7:193–199.

Florijn, B. W., H. van der Graaf, J. W. Schoones, and A. A. Kaptein. 2019. Narrative medicine: A comparison of terminal cancer patients' stories from a Dutch hospice with those of Anatole Broyard and Christopher Hitchens. *Death Studies* 43:570–581.

Frank, A. W. 1991. *At the will of the body: Reflections on illness*. Boston: Houghton Mifflin Company.

Frank, A. W. 1994. Reclaiming an orphan genre: The first-person narrative of illness. *Literature and Medicine* 13:1–21.

Frank, A. W. 1995. *The wounded storyteller. Body, illness, and ethics*. Chicago: The University of Chicago Press.

Frank, A. W. 2007. Five dramas of illness. *Perspectives in Biology and Medicine* 50:379–394.

Frank, A. W. 2010. *Letting stories breathe – a socionarratology*. Chicago: Chicago University Press.

Frank, A. W. 2025. Narrative, experience, and ethics. Illness narrative 2022, unconcluded. Blog Arthur W Frank, June 26.

Frith, H., and D. Harcourt. 2007. Using photographs to capture women's experiences of chemotherapy: Reflecting on the method. *Qualitative Health Research* 17:1340–1350.

Fu, V. X., P. Oomens, V. E. E. Kleinrensink, K. J. Sleurink, W. M. Borst, P. E. Wessels, J. F. Lange, G. J. Kleinrensink, and J. Jeekel. 2020. The effect of preferred music on mental workload and laparoscopic surgical performance in a simulated setting (OPTIMISE): A randomized controlled crossover study. *Surgical Endoscopy* 35:5051–5061.

Gates, H. L., Jr. 1996. White like me. *New Yorker*, 66–81, June 17.

Gibson, C., M. O'Connor, R. White, M. Jackson, S. Baxi, and G. K. B. Halkett. 2022. Silenced: Patients' experiences of voicelessness in head and neck cancer. *Patient Education and Counseling* 105:2410–2416.

Gill, E. 1994. *Le crabe sur la banquette arrière [The crab in the backseat]*. Paris: Mercure de France.

Gray, J.. 2011. Review: Arguably by Christopher Hitchens. *The New Statesman*, October 6.

Grealy, L. 1994. *Autobiography of a face*. Boston: Mariner.

Green, M. J., and K. R. Myers. 2010. Graphic medicine: Use of comics in medical education and patient care. *BMJ* 340:574–577.

Greer, J. A., J. M. Jacobs, A. El-Jawahri, R. J. Nipp, E. R. Gallagher, W. F. Pirl, E. R. Park, A. Muzikansky, J. C. Jacobsen, V. A. Jackson, and J. S. Temel. 2018. Role of patient coping strategies in understanding the effects of early palliative care on quality of life and mood. *Journal of Clinical Oncology* 36:53–60.

von Grueningen, V. E., H. Q. Huang, D. Cella, M. A. Zevon, J. A. LaChance, J. L. Walker, R. Salani, S. C. Modesitt, R. T. Morris, W. H. Bradley, W. P. Boente, L. Wenzel, et al. 2018. Quality of life, symptoms and care needs in patients with persistent or recurrent platinum-resistant ovarian cancer: An NRG Oncology/Gynecologic Oncology Group study. *Gynecologic Oncology* 150:119–126.

Gu, X., X. Shen, J. R. Zhou, J. H. Chu, and L. Jiang. 2024. The effects of common-sense model interventions on cancer patients. A systematic review. *Medicine* 103:17 (e37777).

Gustafsson, L. 1981. *The death of a beekeeper*. New York: New Directions Publ.

Haase, K. R., S. Sattar, S. Hall, B. McLean, A. Wills, et al. 2021. Systematic review of self-management interventions for older adults with cancer. *Psycho-Oncology* 30:989–1008.

Hall, D. 1999. *Without: Poems*. Boston: Mariner.

Hamann, H. A., M. J. Shen, A. J. Thomas, S. J. Craddock Lee, and J. S. Ostroff. 2018a. Development and preliminary psychometric evaluation of a patient-reported outcome measure for lung cancer stigma: The Lung Cancer Stigma Inventory (LCSI). *Stigma Health* 3:195–203.

Hamann, H. A., E. S. Ver Hoeve, L. Carter-Harris, J. L. Studts, and J. S. Ostroff. 2018b. Multilevel opportunities to address lung cancer stigma across the cancer control continuum. *Journal of Thoracic Oncology* 13:1062–1075.

Handler, E. 1996. *Time on fire: My comedy of terrors*. London: Souvenir Press.

Handler, E. 2008. *It's only temporary: The good news and the bad news of being alive*. New York: Riverhead Books.

Hauser, D. J., and N. Schwarz. 2020. The war on prevention II: Battle metaphors undermine cancer treatment and prevention and do not increase vigilance. *Health Communication* 35:1698–1704.

Hawkins, A. H. 1999. *Reconstructing illness – studies in pathography*. West Lafayette: Ind., Purdue University Press.
Hilberdink, K. 2007. *Hans Lodeizen – biografie*. Amsterdam: van Oorschot.
Hitchens, C. 2012. *Mortality*. New York: Twelve.
Hoerni, B. 1994. *Archipel du cancer [Cancer archipelago]*. Paris: La cherche midi éditeur.
Hoerni, B. 2016. Cancer et littérature [Cancer and literature]. *Histoire des Sciences Medicales* 50:199–206.
Hoogerwerf, M. A., M. K. Ninaber, L. N. A. Willems, and A. A. Kaptein. 2012. 'Feelings are facts', Illness perceptions in patients with lung cancer. *Respiratory Medicine* 106:1170–1176.
Howlin, C. 2025. There is more to arts than neural mechanisms: A critique of evidence dismissal in arts and health: Comment on "Can arts-based interventions improve health? A conceptual and methodological critique" by Martin Skov and Marcos Nadal. *Physics of Life Reviews* 54:89–91.
Huang, R. S., D. Chen, A. Benour, R. Cortez, A. Mihalache, C. Johnny, A. Bezjak, R. A. Olson, and S. Raman. 2025. Patient-reported outcomes as prognostic indicators for overall survival in cancer – a systematic review and meta-analysis. *JAMA Oncology*. https://doi.org/10.1001/jamaoncol.2025.3153, in press 11 September 2025.
Hughes, B. M. 2016. *Rethinking psychology: Good science, bad science, pseudoscience*. London: Palgrave.
Hughes, B. M. 2018. *Psychology in crisis*. London: Palgrave.
Hughes, B. 2023. *A conceptual history of psychology: The mind through time*. London: Bloomsbury.
Hughes, B. M. 2025. *Psychology's Quiet Conservatism: How a Supposedly Woke Science Promotes Capitalism and Protects Privilege*. Cham, Switzerland: Palgrave Macmillan.
Hui, D., A. K. Darke, K. A. Guthrie, I. M. Subbiah, J. M. Unger, D. L. Hershman, R. S. Krouse, M. Bakitas, and M. A. O'Rourke. 2022. Association between health-related quality of life and progression-free survival in patients with advanced cancer: A secondary analysis of SWOG clinical trials. *JCO Oncology Practice* 18:e442–e451.
Hunsaker, A. W. 1999. *Reconstructing illness*. West Lafayette: Purdue University Press.
Hutchinson, E. 2001. Book review – *C. Lancet Oncology* 2:321.
Ibuse, M. 1969. *Black rain*. Tokyo: Kodansha Int.
Jansen, F., et al. 2019. Stepped care targeting psychological distress in head and neck cancer and lung cancer patients: Which groups specifically benefit?

Secondary analyses of a randomized trial. *Supportive Care in Cancer* 27:4543–4553.

Jeppesen, E., C. M. Pedersen, K. R. Larsen, E. S. Walsted, A. Rehl, J. Ehrenreich, S. Schnoor, and V. Backer. 2019. Listening to music prior to bronchoscopy reduces anxiety – a randomised controlled trial. *European Clinical Respiratory Journal* 6:1–9.

Jones, T., and K. Pachucki, eds. 2022. *The medical/health humanities – politics, programs, pedagogies*. New York: Springer.

Jones, T., M. Blackie, R. Garden, and D. Wear. 2017. The almost right word: The move from Medical to Health Humanities. *Academic Medicine* 92:932–935.

Jurecic, A. 2012. *Illness as narrative*. Pittsburgh: Pittsburgh University Press.

Kalanithi, P. 2016. *When breath becomes air*. New York: Random House.

Kang, M. C., S. Y. Jung, S. Lee, Y. J. Lee, Y. K. Chung, J. H. Jang, B. Park, and S. Y. Kong. 2025. Causal attributions in patients with breast and gynecological cancers: A scoping review. *Psycho-Oncology* 34:e70253.

Kaplan, R. M. 1990. Behavior as the central outcome in health care. *American Psychologist* 45:1211–1220.

Kaptein, A. A. 2021. Writing cancer. *Supportive Care in Cancer* 29:4375–4380.

Kaptein, A. A. 2022. Novels as data: Health humanities and health psychology. *Journal of Health Psychology* 27:1615–1625.

Kaptein, A. A., and A. C. Lyons. 2010. Cancer ward: Patient perceptions in oncology. *Journal of Health Psychology* 15:848–857.

Kaptein, A. A., and M. S. Y. Thong. 2018. Portraying a grim illness: Lung cancer in novels, poems, films, music, and paintings. *Supportive Cancer Care* 26:3681–3689.

Kaptein, A. A., et al. 2011. Illness perceptions and quality of life in Japanese and Dutch patients with non-small cell lung cancer. *Lung Cancer* 72:384–390.

Kaptein, A. A., A. C. Lyons, A. S. Pearson, S. van der Geest, J. Haan, F. Meulenberg, and J. M. Smyth. 2012. Storying stories. *Medical Education Development* 2:24–26.

Kaptein, A. A., et al. 2013. Illness perceptions and quality of life in Japanese and Dutch women with breast cancer. *Journal of Psychosocial Oncology* 31:83–102.

Kaptein, A. A., B. M. Hughes, M. Murray, and J. M. Smyth. 2018. Start making sense. Art informing health psychology. *Health Psychology Open* 10:1–13.

Kaptein, A. A., J. W. Schoones, P. B. van der Meer, A. Matsuda, M. Murray, L. Heimans, and J. R. Kroep. 2021. Psychosocial determinants of adherence with oral anti- cancer treatment: 'We don't need no education'. *Acta Oncologica* 60:87–95.

Kaptein, A. A., W. E. Hanser, J. W. Schoones, P. Boot, J. W. Pennebaker, and B. M. Hughes. 2025. Cancer in poetry – poetry in cancer: A linguistic analysis of poems by poets on their own cancer and on the cancer of their loved ones. *Psycho-Oncology* 34 (10): e70297.

Kaptein, A. A., J. W. Schoones, Y. M. van der Linden, and B. M. Hughes. Healing beams: Radiation and radiation therapy in novels, poems, music, film, and painting. *Journal of Medical Radiation Sciences* 31:3907–3916.

Karinthy, F. 2006. *A journey round my skull*. New York: New York Review of Books.

Kedia, S. K., et al. 2019. Psychosocial interventions for informal caregivers of lung cancer patients: A systematic review. *Psycho-oncology* 29:251–262.

Kenyon, J. 1996. *Otherwise: New and selected poems*. Minneapolis: Graywolf Press.

Kharade, P., et al. 2018. Appraisal of function after rehabilitation with tongue prosthesis. *Journal of Craniofacial Surgery* 29:e41–e44.

Kim, E., W. Woo, S. Lee, and H. T. Kang. 2025a. Long-term analysis of suicide incidence among patients with lung cancer: A population-based longitudinal study. *Journal of Clinical Medicine* 14:4070.

Kim, M., K. Tan, and L. A. Coombs. 2025b. Effects of web-based interventions on cancer caregivers' burden and quality of life: A systematic review and et-analysis. *Palliative and Supportive Care* 23:e134.

Kleijn, G., B. I. Lissenberg-Witte, E. Bohlmeijer, V. Willemsen, A. Becker-Commissaris, C. M. Eeltink, A. M. E. Bruynzeel, M. J. van der Vorst, P. Cuijpers, and I. M. Verdonck-de Leeuw. 2021. A randomized controlled trial on the efficacy of life review therapy targeting incurably ill cancer patients: Do their informal caregivers benefit? *Supportive Care in Cancer* 29:1257–1264.

Kleinman, A. 1988. *The illness narratives. Suffering, healing, and the human condition*. New York: Basic Books.

Klugman, C. M., and E. G. Lamb, eds. 2019. *Research methods in health humanities*. Oxford: Oxford University Press.

Kluun, R. 2007. *Love life*. London: Pan Books.

Kollaard, S. 2018. *Stage Four*. Seattle: Amazon Crossing.

Körner, A., N. Roberts, R. J. Steele, D. C. Brosseau, and Z. Rosberger. 2019. A randomized controlled trial assessing the efficacy of a self-administered psycho-educational intervention for patients with cancer. *Patient Education and Counseling* 102:735–741.

Lahtinen, A. M., and M. Torppa. 2007. 'Medicalisation of falling in love': Medical students' responses to Thomas Mann's The Black Swan. *Medical Humanities* 33:44–48.

Lambert, S. D., L. O. Brahim, M. Morrison, A. Girgis, M. Yaffe, E. Belzile, K. Clayberg, J. Robinson, S. Thorne, J. L. Bottorff, W. Duggleby, H. Campbell-Enns, K. Youngmee, and C. G. Loiselle. 2019. Priorities for caregiver research in cancer care: An international Delphi survey of caregivers, clinicians, managers, and researchers. *Supportive Care in Cancer* 27:805–817.

Lawrence, C., T. Mhlaba, K. A. Stewart, R. Moletsane, B. Gaede, and M. Moshabela. 2018. The hidden curricula of medical education: A scoping review. *Academic Medicine* 93:648–656.

Lawson, D. 2001. Introduction. In *Snake oil and other preoccupations*, ed. J. Diamond. London: Vintage.

Lefkovits, Y. R., N. Heriot, A. Sporik, S. Perera, M. Friedlander, C. Dixon, et al. 2024. Incorporating patient-reported outcome measures (PROMs) into a clinical quality registry (CQR) for ovarian cancer: Considerations and challenges. *BMC Health Services Research* 24:778.

Leibovitz, A. 2006. *A photographers' life 1990–2005*. New York: Random House.

Leventhal, H. 2019. Next steps for examining the common-sense of health behaviour. *Health Psychology Review* 13:487–489.

Leventhal, H., L. A. Phillips, and E. Burns. 2016. The Common-Sense Model of Self-Regulation: A dynamic framework for understanding illness self-management. *Journal of Behavioral Medicine* 39:935–946.

Levinsen, A. K. G, S. O. Dalton, E. Jakobsen, I. Gögenur, M. Borre, and R. Zachariae, et al. In Press. Prevalence of and factors associated with clinically important levels of fatigue, pain, and insomnia in survivors of cancer: A population-based cross-sectional study. *Journal of Cancer Survivorship*.

Linklater, A.. 2012. Mortality by Christopher Hitchens: Review. *The Observer*, August 26.

Liu, F., H. Shan, W. Bing, L. Sun, and L. Wei. 2025. Relationship between symptom burden and benefit finding in patients with gastrointestinal cancers undergoing chemotherapy: The chain-mediating role of comprehensive needs and communication pattern. *Supportive Care in Cancer* 33:816.

Ljunggren, B. 1993. Herbert Olivecrona: Founder of Swedish neurosurgery. *Journal of Neurosurgery* 78:142–149.

Lodeizen, H. 1966. *Poems [Het innerlijk behang]*. Amsterdam: van Oorschot.

Lo-Fo-Wong, D., A. Beijaerts, H. C. J. M. de Haes, and M. A. G. Sprangers. 2014. Cancer in full-colour: Use of a graphic novel to identify distress in women with breast cancer. *Journal of Health Psychology* 19:1554–1563.

Lorde, A. 1983. There is no hierarchy of oppressions. *Interracial Books for Children Bulletin* 14 (3–4): 9.

Lorde, A. 1997. *The cancer journals*. San Francisco: Aunt Lute Books.

Łuczyk, R. J., K. Sikora, A. Bodio, M. Łuczyk, M. Baryła-Matejczuk, A. Wawryniuk, et al. 2024. Role of emotional control on anxiety and stress among cancer patients. *Cancer Medicine* 13:e70162.

Mäkitie, A. A., R. O. Alabi, L. Pulkki-Råback, A. Almangush, J. J. Beitler, N. F. Saba, et al. 2024. Psychological factors related to treatment outcomes in head and neck cancer. *Advances in Therapy* 41:3489–3519.

Malibiran, R., J. D. Tariman, and Amer K. Bibliotherapy. 2018. Appraisal of evidence for patients diagnosed with cancer. *Clinical Journal of Oncology Nursing* 22:377–380.

Mann, T. 1993. *The black swan*. Berkeley: University of California Press.

Maomai, M. 1997. *Krebs schreiben [Writing cancer]*. Mannheim: Röhrig Universitätsverlag.

Marchetto, M. A. 2006. *Cancer Vixen*. New York: Knopfler.

Marsman, L. 2019. *The following scan will last five minutes*. Liverpool: Liverpool University Press.

McCullers, C. 1998. *Clock without hands*. Boston: Houghton Mifflin Co.

McCurry, J. 2015. Hiroshima survivors remember. *Lancet* 386:417–418.

McMullin, J. 2016. Cancer and the Comics: Graphic narratives and biolegitimate lives. *Medical Anthropology Quarterly* 30:149–167.

McNeil, C. M. 2018. Grace and forgiveness. *Journal of Clinical Oncology* 36:1045–1046.

Merz, E. L., R. S. Fox, and V. L. Malcarne. 2014. Expressive writing interventions in cancer patients: A systematic review. *Health Psychology Review* 8:339–361.

Miller, M., M. Meyers, K. Krainak, and S. P. Lewis. 2025. Interventions to support spirituality among adults with cancer: A scoping review. *Supportive Care in Cancer* 33:742.

Miranda, K. W., B. L. Musher, and H. J. Badr. 2025. Unmet supportive care needs in patients with advanced cancer and its impact on distress. *BMC Palliative Care* 24:110.

Mische, Lawson L., J. Cline, A. French, and N. Ismael. 2017. Patient perceptions of a 1-h art-making experience during blood and marrow transplant treatment. *European Journal of Cancer Care* 26:1–10.

Moreno-Alonso, D., B. G. García, C. Madrid-Alejos, G. Morón-Cazalilla, S. Llorens-Torromé, I. Crespo, et al. 2025. Bridging the gap: An updated systematic integrative review of palliative care integration in hematological malignancies. *Seminars in Oncology Nursing* xxx:151962.

Moser, B. 2019. *Sontag – her life*. New York: Harper Collins.

Naef, A. P., and E. William. 1998. Adams: Thomas Mann and The Magic Mountain. *Annals of Thoracic Surgery* 65:285–287.

Naghshineh, S., J. P. Hafler, A. R. Miller, M. A. Blanco, S. R. Lipsitz, R. P. Dubroff, S. Khoshbin, and J. T. Katz. 2008. Formal art observation training improves medical students' visual diagnostic skills. *Journal of General Internal Medicine* 2:991–997.

Naono, A. 2019. The origins of 'Hibakusha' as a scientific and political classification of the survivor. *Japanese Studies* 39:333–352.

Nijhoff, G. 2018. *Sickness work*. Singapore: Palgrave.

Niscola, P., D. Piccioni, and M. Giovannini. 2025. Palliative care interventions and their early integration in the management of older adults with acute myeloid leukaemia: A narrative review. *Annals of Palliative Medicine* 14:393–411.

Nisiraiou, A., A. Bozas, D. Kyrou, K. Stavrogianni, M. M. Vasilopoulou, G. M. Kalomoiris, et al. 2025. Post-traumatic growth in adult cancer survivors: A scoping review of psychological factors, predictors, and interventions. *International Journal of Psychiatry* 60:e70097.

Nogueria, C. M., B. S. Reis, A. de F. R. Meneses, B. H. Mellado, and Reis FJC. 2025. Unveiling delays: Understanding the diagnostic pathways of women with advanced cervical cancer. *Supportive Care in Cancer* 33:826.

O'Mahony, S. 2013. Against narrative medicine. *Perspectives in Biology and Medicine* 56:611–619.

Oates J. C. 2017. The poet of freakiness. *New York Review of Books*, September 28, 78–80.

Ogden, J. 2023. *Health psychology*. London: McGrawHill.

Olson, L. 2011. Anger among allies: Audre Lorde's 1981 keynote admonishing the National Women's Studies Association. *Quarterly Journal of Speech* 97 (3): 283–308.

Orr, L. D., J. Vanderpoel, P. Vadagam, M. I. Patel, U. B. Roy, B. Ledezma, et al. 2025. Patient, care partner, and provider voice in treatment decision-making for non-small cell lung cancer. *Patient Education and Counseling* 136:108776.

Ousager, J., and H. Johannessen. 2010. Humanities in undergraduate medical education: A literature review. *Academic Medicine* 85:988–998.

Paulson, A. E., A. Stein, J. K. Kendal, N. M. Bernthal, and L. E. Wessel. 2024. Most patients with bone sarcomas seek emotional support and information about other patients' experiences: A thematic analysis. *Clinical Orthopedic Related Research* 482:161–171.

Peabody, F. 2009. Toward a restorative medicine – the science of care. *JAMA* 301: 1710–1712 [JAMA, 1927, 88, 877–882].

Pelosi, A. J. 2019. Personality and fatal diseases: Revisiting a scientific scandal. *Journal of Health Psychology* 24:421–439.

Pennebaker, J. W., and J. F. Evans. 2014. *Expressive writing: Words that heal.* Bedford, Indiana: Idyll Arbor.

Pereira, N. R. P., S. J. Janssen, N. Stoop, S. Hartvelt, Y. Chen, T. F. DeLaney, F. J. Hornicek, and J. H. Schwab. 2019. Physical function and quality of life after resection of mobile spine chondrosarcoma. *Global Spine Journal* 9:743–753.

Philipp, R., A. Mehnert, C. Lo, V. Mueler, M. Reck, and S. Vehling. 2019. Characterizing death acceptance among patients with cancer. *Psycho-Oncology* 28:854–862.

Pils, S., J. Ott, A. Reinthaller, E. Steiner, S. Springer, and R. Ristl. 2020. Effect of viewing Disney movies during chemotherapy on self-reported quality of life among patients with gynecologic cancer. *JAMA Network Open* 3:1–10.

Porter, L. S., G. Samsa, J. L. Steel, L. C. Hanson, T. W. LeBlanc, J. Bull, S. Fischer, and F. J. Keefe. 2019. Caregiver-guided pain coping skills training for patients with advanced cancer: Background, design, and challenges for the CaringPals study. *Clinical Trials* 16:262–272.

Post, K. E., S. Aribindi, L. Traeger, D. Hall, J. Jacobs, J. S. Temel, et al. 2025. Not out of the woods: Perspectives from patients with triple-negative breast cancer. *Supportive Care in Cancer* 33:18.

Price, R. 1994. *A whole new life: An illness and a healing*. New York: Atheneum.

Rabow, M. W., S. Goodman, S. Chang, M. Berger, and S. Folkman. 2010. Filming the family: A documentary film to educate clinicians about family caregivers of patients with brain tumors. *Journal of Cancer Education* 25:242–246.

Richardson, E. M., N. Schüz, K. Sanderson, J. L. Scott, and B. Schüz. 2017. Illness representations, coping, and illness outcomes in people with cancer: A systematic review and meta-analysis. *Psycho-Oncology* 26:724–737.

Richardson, A. E., E. Broadbent, and R. P. Morton. 2019. A systematic review of psychological interventions for patients with head and neck cancer. *Supportive Care in Cancer* 27:2007–2021.

Rieff, D. 2008. *Swimming in a sea of death: A son's memoir*. New York: Simon & Schuster.

Riskin, J. 2016. *The restless clock: A history of the centuries-long argument over what makes living things tick*. Chicago: University of Chicago Press.

Rodin, G., E. An, J. Shnall, and C. Malfitano. 2020. Psychological interventions for patients with advanced disease: Implications for oncology and palliative care. *Journal of Clinical Oncology* 38:885–904.

Romagna, A., C. Schwartz, B. Huffman, W. Hitzl, R. A. Kristof, H. Clusmann, and C. Blume. 2025. Analysis of quality of life and outcomes of vestibular schwannoma patients after resection and radiosurgery in an interdisciplinary treatment concept. *Nature Scientific Reports* 15:15941.

Roth, P. 1991. *Patrimony*. New York: Vintage Books.

Ruben, M. A., D. Blanch-Hartigan, and J. C. Shipherd. 2018. To know another's pain: A meta-analysis of caregivers' and healthcare providers' pain assessment accuracy. *Annals of Behavioral Medicine* 52:662–685.

Rueb, M., M. Siebeck, E. A. Rehfuess, and L. M. Pfadenhauer. 2022. Cinemeducation in medicine: A mixed methods study on students' motivations and benefits. *BMC Medical Education* 22:172.

Sabin, R. 1996. *Comics, Comix & Graphic Novels*. New York: Phaidon Press.

Sain, A. M. de, C. Ruis, M. L. Zomers, M. E. G. ten Hoor-Suykerbuyk, T. Kuunders, F. Y. F. L. de Vos, A. Janssens, and T. Seute. 2025. Towards a definition of an existential approach in cancer patients: A co-produced scoping review. *PLOS One* 20 (9): e0330384.

Samuel J. N., Booth, C. M., Eisenhauer, E., Brundage, M., Berry, S. R., and Gyawali, B. 2022. Association of quality-of-life outcomes in cancer drug trials with survival outcomes and drug class. *JAMA Oncolology* 1:879–886.

Sánchez-Gómez, C., E. J. Fernández-Rodriguez, S. Jiménez-Sánchez, E. Fonseca-Sánchez, J. Perez, V. Navarro-López, et al. 2025. Effect of cognitive training on cancer-related cognitive impairment in patients with breast cancer: A systematic review and meta-analysis. *Psycho-Oncology* 34:e70251.

Scalman, M. 2015. *Poetry in medicine*. New York: Persea Books.

Schmidt, N. 2018a. *The wounded self*. Rochester N.Y: Camden House.

Schmidt, N. 2018b. Intertextuality and the transnational in Verena Stefan's Fremdschläfer (2007): Writing breast cancer from beyond the border. In *The wounded self, writing illness in twenty-first-century German literature*, ed. N. Schmidt, 92–113. Rochester NY: Camden House.
Sisi, Y., C. Yao, K. Yajuan, S. Suting, J. Du, H. Qu, et al. 2025. Pulmonary rehabilitation for patients receiving lung cancer radiotherapy: A scoping review. *BMJ Open* 15:e091749.
Skov, M., and M. Nadal. 2025. Can arts-based interventions improve health? A conceptual and methodological critique. *Physics of Life Reviews* 53:239–259.
Slawson, D. C., and A. F. Shaughnessy. 1997. Obtaining useful information from expert based sources. *BMJ* 314:947–953.
Snow, C. P. 1964. *The two cultures*. Cambridge: Cambridge University Press.
Solzhenitsyn, A. 1968. *Cancer ward*. Harmondsworth: Penguin.
Sonke J, M. K. B. Tan, J. B. Lee, V. Pesata, A. Akram, T. Golden, et al. 2025. The arts for disease prevention and health promotion: A systematic review. *Nature Medicine* 31:3907–3916.
Sontag, S. 1978. *Illness as metaphor*. New York: Farrar, Straus Giroux.
Sowell, F. G., T. de Milliano, K. J. S. Brady, G. Foglia, M. Sasane, S. Bensfia, et al. 2025. A conceptual model for advanced/metastatic gastric or gastroesophageal junction cancer: A review of qualitative studies and results from patient interviews. *BMC Cancer* 25:88.
Staples, B. 2003. Editorial observer; back when skin color was destiny–unless you passed for white. *New York Times*, September 7.
Stefan, V. 2007. *Alien sleepers*. Zurich: Ammann Verlag.
Strawson, G. 2004. Against narrativity. *Ratio* 17:428–452.
Subramanian, R., and M. J. Brooks. 2022. How a medical orchestra cultivates creativity, joy, empathy, and connection. *AMA Journal of Ethics* 24 (7): E584–E589.
Swain, K. 2017. Podcast: The Chemo files: One year on. *Lancet Oncology* 18:179.
Tang, M., X. Liu, Q. Wu, and Y. Shi. 2020. The effects of cognitive-behavioral stress management for breast cancer patients. *Cancer Nursing* 43:222–237.
Temel, J., J. A. Greer, A. Muzikansky, E. R. Gallagher, S. Admane, V. A. Jackson, C. M. Dahlin, C. D. Blindermann, J. Jacobsen, W. F. Pirl, J. A. Billings, and T. J. Lynch. 2010. Early palliative care for patients with metastatic non-small-cell lung cancer. *New England Journal of Medicine* 363:733–742.
Terayama, T., J. Shigemura, Y. Kobayashi, M. Kurosawa, M. Nagamine, H. Toda, et al. 2021. Mental health consequences for survivors of the 2011

Fukushima nuclear disaster: A systematic review. Part 2: Emotional and behavioral consequences. *CNS Spectrums* 26:30–42.
Timmermann, C. 2014. *A history of lung cancer. The recalcitrant disease.* New York: Palgrave.
Tolstoy, L. N. 2010. *The death of Ivan Ilyich.* Seattle: Pacific Publishers Studio.
Trigueros-Murillo, A., J. Martinez-Calderon, M. J. Casuso-Holgado, P. González-García, and A. M. Heredia-Rizo. 2023. Effects of music-based interventions on cancer-related pain, fatigue, and distress: An overview of systematic reviews. *Supportive Care in Cancer* 31:488.
Tsiakiri, A., A. Despoti, P. Koutsimani, K. Megari, S. Plakias, and A. Tsapanou. 2025. Mapping cognitive oncology: A decade of trends and research fronts. *Medical Sciences* 13:19.
Tundealao, S., P. Okunlola, O. Alabaku, O. Noah, O. Alufa, and T. Titiloye. 2025. Head and neck related quality of life following glossectomy among tongue cancer patients: A systematic review and meta-analysis. *Oral and Maxillofacial Surgery* 29:164.
Turkman, Y. E., H. P. Kennedy, L. N. Harris, and M. T. Knobf. 2016. 'An addendum to breast cancer': The triple negative experience. *Supportive Care in Cancer* 24:3715–3721.
Twiddy, I. 2015. *Cancer poetry.* Basingstoke: Palgrave Macmillan.
Updike, J. 1982. From the journal of a leper. *American Journal of Dermatopathology* 4:137–142.
Vanistendael, J. 2012. *When David Lost His Voice.* London: SelfMadeHero.
Vega, S. 2016. *Lover, beloved.* Amanuensis: CD.
Verghese, A. 2020. Writing medicine. *JAMA* 323:1649–1650.
Vestdijk, S. 1964. *De zieke mens in de romanliteratuur [The ill person in literature].* Delft: Koninklijke Nederlandse Gist – en Spiritusfabriek.
Watson, J., C. S. Peng, M. Desir, M. N. Mate-Cole, and H. Amonoo. 2025. Expressive writing interventions in patients with cancer: A scoping literature review. *Palliative and Supportive Care* 23 (e132): 1–20.
Whitt, J. 1999. The "we of me": Carson McCullers as lesbian novelist. *Journal of Homosexuality* 37:127–139.
Wijdicks, E. F. M. 2020. *Cinema MD – a history of medicine on screen.* Oxford: Oxford University Press.
Williams, I. C. M. 2012. Graphic medicine: Comics as medical narrative. *Medical Humanities* 38:21–27.
Wong, L. 2012. *Scales to scalpels: Doctors who practice in the healing arts of music and medicine.* New York: Pegasus.

Wong, S. S., T. J. George, M. Godfrey, J. Le, and D. B. Pereira. 2019. Using photography to explore psychological distress in patients with pancreatic cancer and their caregivers: A qualitative study. *Supportive Care in Cancer* 27:321–328.

Woolf, V. 1930. *On being ill*. London: The Hogarth Press.

Wu, T. J., C. S. Sheih, S. T. Jou, C. Y. Lee, T. Y. Yu, C. Y. Liu, and C. W. Chen. 2025. Effects of bibliotherapy on emotional distress, coping strategies, and resilience in adolescents with cancer: A pilot randomized controlled trial. *European Journal of Oncology Nursing* 76:102900.

Xiang, J., L. Dai, L. Tan, D. Lv, Y. Chen, L. Tang, et al. 2025. Psychosocial experiences of prostate cancer survivors after treatment: A systematic review of qualitative studies. *Frontiers in Public Health* 13:1625611.

Zhang, Y., X. Chen, R. Li, Y. Wang, Z. Sun, and Q. Li. 2024. Interventions strategies and their efficacy in illness perceptions in patients with cancer: A systematic review and meta-analysis. *European Journal of Oncology Nursing* 70:102599.

Zorn, F. 1979. *Mars*. Frankfurt an Main: Fischer Taschen Verlag.

Zulman, D. M., M. C. Haverfield, J. G. Shaw, C. G. Brown-Johnson, R. Schwartz, A. A. Tierney, D. L. Zionts, N. Safaeinili, M. Fischer, Israni S. Thadaney, S. M. Asch, and A. Verghese. 2020. Practices to foster physician presence and connection with patients in the clinical encounter. *JAMA* 323:70–81.

Index[1]

[1] Note: Page numbers followed by 'n' refer to notes.

A. A. Kaptein, B. M. Hughes, *Writing Cancer*,
https://doi.org/10.1007/978-981-95-6501-6